THE STATIN DAMAGE CRISIS

Duane Graveline, M.D., M.P.H.

THE STATIN DAMAGE CRISIS
By Duane Graveline, M.D., M.P.H.

With introduction by
Malcolm Kendrick, MD

Copyright 2012 by Duane Graveline, M.D., M.P.H.

The Statin Damage Crisis
Third Edition: July 2012

ISBN 978-1-4243-3869-6

PUBLISHED BY: Duane Graveline, M.D., M.P.H.

The information and opinions in this book are based upon the author's personal and professional experiences and research. Information in this book is not intended to be a substitute for professional medical advice and care. Always consult with a qualified medical professional before making medication, supplement, or lifestyle changes or decisions.

Duane Graveline, M.D., M.P.H.

ACKNOWLEDGEMENT

To all my friends and colleagues in the medical, health, nutrition and research professions whose knowledge and guidance have paved the way to my writing this book, my gratitude is endless. Your encouragement and advice were essential ingredients to its becoming.

But the most profound encouragement for my bringing these unknown and often obscure cognitive, neuromuscular and behavioral side effects of the statin drugs to public attention comes from the letters and e-mails I have received from thousands of patients, their families and concerned friends, here in the U.S.A and around the world. Their almost desperate need to understand what has happened or was happening to them and why was a powerful incentive— especially in the denial or ignorance of these many different side effects by their doctors and other health caregivers. So many of these victims have related how learning about my experience with transient global amnesia has helped relieve the stress and anxiety about their own concerns. I hope this book fulfills their expectations for more complete information about the true legacy of statin drugs as currently used and guidance towards alternative therapies, when indicated.

Duane Graveline, M.D., M.P.H.

CONTENTS

Introduction by Malcolm Kendrick, MD – Page 9

Foreword – Page 13

1.How Statin Drugs Work - Page 17

2.Mevalonate Blockade - Page 35

3.Statins and Brain Cholesterol - Page 39

4.Statins and CoQ10 - Page 43

5.Statins and Dolichols - Page 49

6.Statins and Nuclear Factor-*kappa* B - Page 53

7.The Role of Cholesterol in the Body - Page 57

8.Inflammation and Atherosclerosis - Page 63

9.The Misguided War on Cholesterol - Page 71

10. A Failed National Diet.What Diet Then? – Page 79

11. Enter Glyconutrients – Page 87

12. Anti-Inflammatory Alternatives to Statins – Page 93
a.) Omegas 3 and 6 – Page 95
b.) Ubiquinol, the CoQ10 of choice – Page 98
c.) Tocotrienols, the New Vitamin E – Page 99
d.) Aged Garlic Extract (AGE) – Page 102
e.) Vitamin D – Page 103
f.) Low Dose Statins – Page 105
g.) Red Yeast Rice – Page 106
h.) Diet – Page 106

CONTENTS CONTINUED

13. Failure of MedWatch – Page 107
Adverse Drug Reports for Lipitor 1997 to 2012 – Page110

14. Serious Statin Drug Side Effects – Page 117
a.) The ALS / Statin Link – Page 117
b.) Permanent Peripheral Neuropathy – Page 120
c.) Permanent Myopathy – Page 121
d.) Chronic Neuromuscular Degeneration - Page 124

15. Mitochondrial Mutations – Page 129
1.) CoQ10 – Page 132
2.) Vitamin C – Page 132
3.) Selenium – Page 135
4.) Glyconutrients – Page 136
5.) Lecithin – Page 137
6.) Omegas 3 & 6 – Page 138
7.) Tocopherol Vitamin E – Page 142
8.) Tocotrienol Vitamin E – Page 143
9.) Magnesium – Page 144
10.) L- Carnitine – Page 144
11.) Alpha Lipoic Acid – Page 145
12.) Vitamin D – Page 146
13.) D-ribose – Page 148

16. My Personal Statin Experience - Page 151

17. Conclusion – Page 163

Appendices.
A.) FDA Expands List of Statin Precautions – Page 167
B.) Causes of Statin Side Effects – Page 171

References – Page 175

Introduction by Malcolm Kendrick MD
'Statins don't do that.'

The medical world in thrall to statins. They are the 'wonder drug.' Many doctors believe that everyone in the world should be taking a statin. Some suggest children as young as eight should start on statins, and take them for the rest of their lives. These are drugs with enormous benefit, and are virtually side-effect free. That, at least is the current dogma. To criticize statins is to be cast to the outer darkness of scientific medical debate.

The reality is that statins are extremely potent drugs which interfere with our body biochemistry at a very fundamental level. They block the production of—not just cholesterol; in itself a critical substance that is essential for human life and health. They also block the production of other vital chemicals; co-enzyme Q-10 and dolichols, to name but two.

Most doctors have never heard of these substances, they have no idea what they do, and have not the slightest idea that statins interfere with their production. Yet, these are vital chemicals that are used throughout the body in a myriad of different ways. (Try asking your doctor what a dolichol is, and await the blank look.)

The body is clever enough to bypass problems with a few vital chemicals—at least for a while. In the end, however, after you have poisoned our biochemistry for long enough, problems will emerge. Problems, for example, with thinking and remembering. These are a direct result of blocking cholesterol production.

The synapses in our brains—that allow you to form memories—include pure cholesterol. Yet doctors dismiss reports of memory problems with statins, mainly because they can't see how a statin could have this effect. Yes, folks, what do they teach people at medical school?

Muscle pains, tiredness, weakness. These too are a direct result of blocking co-enzyme Q-10 production. This is an enzyme vital to energy production in cells. Depression, irritability, mood swings. These are commonly seen with statins. They are a direct result of blocking dolichol production.

Duane Graveline has done the world a great service by gathering together thousands of reports of statin drug side-effects. These range from minor muscle pains, to the complete destruction of muscles, kidney failure then death. They include the very worrying possibility that statins may accelerate, or even cause, Lou Gehrig's disease (Amyotrophic Lateral Sclerosis - ALS). And that is just for starters. On the horizon lies cancer.

My own view is that everyone who takes a statin will suffer side-effects. Some are very minor, some are highly significant. The one thing likely to be the same for all reported side-effects is that they are universally dismissed by doctors. Doctors who have been brain-washed into believing that statins are 'side-effect free wonder drugs.' 'Statins don't do that' is their battle cry when anyone dares mention a side-effect. Even side-effects that are listed by the drug manufacturers themselves.

Duane Graveline himself suffered transient global amnesia whilst taking statins. What was he told? 'Statins don't do that.' Sorry you misguided medical fools. Statins do that. They also cause depression, and trigger violent and impulsive behaviour.

The tragedy here is that we have statins. The most widely prescribed drugs in the history of mankind—by a distance. Yet none of the drug safety organisation around the world has ever set up a proper study on the effects of these drugs in the general population.

We are told that the adverse event reporting system will reveal any problems, if they exist. This is complete nonsense. At very best adverse event reporting picks up 1 to 5% of actual problems, and these would be the very systems that failed to notice any problems at all with VIOXX®. A drug estimated to have killed fifty to one hundred thousand people in the USA alone, in three years.

The reality is that these systems don't work. They can't even detect a massive surge in deaths caused by a drug, let alone non-fatal side-effects. They especially don't pick up on side-effects that are not listed by the manufacturer in the first place.

If you are taking a statin drug, you owe it to yourself to read this book. Maybe it won't change your mind. The world has, after all, been trained to be terrified of cholesterol levels and you probably believe that you will die if you don't take your statin. This is complete and utter nonsense, of course.

Even taking the best possible figures, from selected trials, and painting them in the best possible light. If you took a statin for thirty years, you could expect five to six months of increased life expectancy. And that's it. And that is only for men, with pre-existing heart disease. For women, forget it. These drugs are pointless, and cannot extend your life by one day.

But, hey, if you want to believe the hype....For everyone else, read this book. You will be doing yourself a massive favour. Thank you Duane for having the courage to fight against the statin insanity that has gripped the world.

Malcolm Kendrick MD
(Author of *The Great Cholesterol Con*)

FOREWORD

Pharmageddon

The term Pharmageddon seems created specifically for the marketing of statins. Look at the facts!

Forty years ago Ancel Keys sold the concept of cholesterol etiology of cardiovascular disease to the powers that be in Washington and the war was on—the misguided war on cholesterol. Starting in the mid-fifties anyone walking counter-current to this philosophy was considered ill-informed and seriously behind the times. I wrote thousands of prescriptions for whatever cholesterol buster was in vogue at the time. I lectured at high schools, men's clubs and to each of my sometimes skeptical patients on the evils of eggs, whole milk and butter. I raised my family on no eggs, skim milk and margarine, so convinced I was that for every 1% of cholesterol lowering, we would gain two more years of productive life. Like all of my peers I was riding the anti-cholesterol bandwagon. Who wouldn't? You give cholesterol to rabbits, they get atherosclerosis. You take cholesterol away, the atherosclerosis disappears. What more proof did you need?

Suddenly in the mid-fifties we had this new disease, that of cholesterol elevation, and millions of people were dying unnecessarily from heart disease and strokes. Very few people had the slightest doubt about the information base on which this imposing cholesterol edifice was erected. None of us realized that Keys had consciously manipulated the data to include only those studies that agreed with his preconceived idea. None of us was scientist enough to know the difference between natural cholesterol of angelic disposition and its devilish oxy-cholesterol brother that blocked rabbit arteries with such ease. All of us were looking for better ways to lower cholesterol. Well meaning researchers would spend their lives trying to sort out which of the many lipid components floating about our blood stream was the biggest enemy. We were delighted when drug company scientists discovered the reductase step along the biochemical path to cholesterol synthesis. Suddenly we had a meaningful weapon.

We had been chipping away at cholesterol for 30 years without doing much good. We needed that big gun and the billion dollar statin industry was on! None of us even bothered to look in our dusty textbooks to find out just where this reductase step was located and what things other than cholesterol might be involved when we knocked over that one domino. Merck had a few good men then and they even filed for a CoQ10 patent so they could combine their Zocor with CoQ10 but then decided no one else was bothering so why should they. That should have aroused our suspicions then but it didn't. Looking back on all this, I still feel very uncomfortable at how completely naive I was but in those days we all seemed to trust the drug companies as working for us. I was no different from my peers.

Not only were we as doctors convinced but we had the whole world convinced that cholesterol was our enemy. We could use the cholesterol word to frighten small children. Within only a few years, millions of people were on statins. A few had unusual reactions. Some of those, including myself, started to really research these statins, suspecting the drug companies had not done their job adequately or might have tweaked the data just a bit. We were right on both counts but how to tell the world? Media kings were paid princely sums for carrying their statin ads and editors were well aware which side of the bread was buttered. After their drug company grooming, our doctors, hopelessly antagonistic to cholesterol, predictably reacted *en bloc* to the possibility of serious problems with their favorite drug. They dismissed every bad word their hapless patients related to them, since they had been told nothing by their formal processes of physician education. Of course not! The drug companies had the FDA in their pocket and the doctors were being informed by young "drug reps" each carefully trained to say only what they were supposed to say. Billions of dollars were at stake.

It would have been smart to look into the whole statin side effect issue then but we didn't. Only in the past few years has the true legacy of statins emerged and it is no wonder that doctors do not care to look at it.

Then came news about cholesterol's possible irrelevance. Statins worked, it was discovered, not by cholesterol reduction but by their powerful anti-inflammatory action[1]. Atherosclerosis was an inflammatory process and the proper treatment now was anti-inflammation. Study after study proved this effect of statins. They worked better than anything else we had for vascular inflammation and could be used successfully for almost anything having an inflammatory component.

Our cholesterol disease was rapidly disappearing. In its place was rising a new edifice to the role of inflammation. How best to handle this confusing fact from the viewpoint of the drug industry? — pretend it isn't happening! Keep the doctors focused on cholesterol as long as we can, for billions of dollars are at stake and if we play our cards right we might slide cholesterol out and inflammation in and never miss a statin sale. As to the side effects of statins, we will pretend we do not hear about them. After all we do control the communication channels.

This is where I find myself today after twelve years of investigating the side effects of statin drugs. Although I have amassed volumes of carefully referenced information supporting my concerns, the great majority of the physicians out there today are just like I was, proudly riding the anti-cholesterol bandwagon, confident that statins are the best drug we have and bowing to every whim of the FDA and the drug companies. Who am I to be critical of our institutions? So I have given up my allegiance to cholesterol and the statins, does that make me better than my peers? No, just better informed, I murmur quietly trying to understand why after all these years of working to inform, the average doctor's philosophy about cholesterol and statins is unchanged and all they seem to know about statin side effects is that, "Statins may cause a few aches and pains and occasional liver inflammation"– exactly what I was told many years ago when I was a practicing physician. I shake my head sadly. That is not progress.

Duane Graveline MD MPH
Author of: *Lipitor*[R]*, Thief of Memory*, *Statin Drugs Side Effects, and the Misguided War on Cholesterol,* and *The Dark Side of Statins.*

CHAPTER 1
How Statin Drugs Work

The development of statin drugs was an almost inevitable phenomenon. After decades of concentrating on cholesterol as the supposed culprit in arteriosclerosis and atherosclerosis, the pharmaceutical community wasn't about to waste its time and resources looking for anything except the simplest way to "cut it off at the pass."

The biogenesis of cholesterol starts from a simple chemical reaction: Under the influence of ultraviolet radiation, photosynthetic plants combine water with carbon dioxide, the well-known gas we exhale in every breath, to form glucose, the fuel of our bodies.

From this humble origin, the first step toward production of cholesterol in the human body involves the process of glycolysis in which glucose is converted into the two-carbon building blocks of life known as Acetyl-CoA. These simple fragments then combine to start the cholesterol biosynthetic pathway. Next, three molecules of Acetyl-CoA combine stepwise to form the six-carbon hydroxymethyl glutaric acid part of the intermediate complex known as HMG-CoA, which has proven to be the Achilles heel of cholesterol biosynthesis.

This is the weak point in the chain of events the pharmaceutical industry was looking for and the one that enabled them to develop their statin drugs, for when two molecules of HMG-CoA next combined to form the ubiquitous mevalonic acid, the enzyme, HMG-CoA reductase was required. This enzyme was quite easily inhibited and suddenly a multibillion-dollar industry was born with the development of the HMG-CoA reductase inhibitors known as the statin drugs. Whether Lipitor®, Mevacor®, Zocor®, Pravachol®, Crestor®, Lescol®, Livalo® or the ill-fated Baycol®, all use the same mechanism and are merely variations of the same theme as marketed by different pharmaceutical companies to obtain market share.

Research biochemists soon identified the HMG-CoA reductase step as a natural control point for cholesterol synthesis since the reaction was not reversible and it was the slowest step of the entire cholesterol pathway. It seemed a natural point for cholesterol control—the pharmaceutical companies now had their "corral." One can almost feel the pulse of industry leaders quicken in anticipation of the potential market size.

Cholesterol, discovered as a major constituent of gallstones, was isolated in 1784 as the first known steroid. Its exact chemical structure was found only in 1932 after 70 years of active research. As a steroid, it is a member of the vast array of natural products known as the terpenoids. Man has used these substances since antiquity as ingredients of flavors, preservatives, perfumes, medicines, narcotics, soaps and pigments. By 1894 the name terpene was derived from research into the manufacture of camphor from turpentine. The relationship of steroids to the terpenoids was not discovered until the late 1950's. Since then the modern study of cholesterol has included some of the most creative and productive scientists of the twentieth century. The biosynthesis of cholesterol was worked out by the biochemists Konrad Bloch, Rudolph Schoenheimer, Fyodor Lynen and many others. Bloch, who received the Nobel Prize in 1964, was Kilmer McCully's mentor at Harvard, helping to guide the promising young biochemist and beginning pathologist along his future path of elucidating homocysteine's role in the etiology of arteriosclerosis. The research on the biosynthesis of cholesterol continues undiminished today. Scientists marvel at the astonishing efficiency and sheer elegance of the steroid biosynthetic pathway. Its complexity is such as to nearly defy human credulity.

The mevalonic acid-HMG-CoA reductase step is but the first step on the long climb to cholesterol synthesis. Many intermediate steps are required before the ultimate goal of cholesterol synthesis is achieved. Statin drugs, while curtailing cholesterol biosynthesis, must inevitably inhibit the production of these vital intermediary products, primary among which are ubiquinone (coenzyme Q10)[1] and dolichols. One might say these unavoidable, collateral consequences might yet prove to be the Achilles heel of the statin drugs in that the side effects resulting from impaired production of these substances are intolerable, harmful and even lethal to many people.

The pharmaceutical industry has long been attempting to develop a means by which interference with cholesterol production might be achieved farther along the biosynthetic pathway, beyond the point where these vital intermediary products originate, but up to now have failed. There is reason to believe that such biochemical maneuvering, even if successful for restoring such vital intermediary substances as ubiquinone and dolichols, may be completely inadequate to address the full spectrum of physiological consequences from statin drug use. Certainly any hormonal consequences from inadequate cholesterol availability, such as testosterone and progesterone deficiency, would remain an issue. And, as Pfreiger has so brilliantly demonstrated, impairment of synapse formation and function in our brain cells from deficient cholesterol manufacture by our glial cells would continue unabated. Additionally, even if the dedicated researchers of the pharmaceutical industry discover a way around these two very substantial side effects, even greater hurdles exist from recent evidence that statins work not by cholesterol manipulation but by some basic anti-inflammatory role. [2,3,4,5,6]

Key to this is a substance known as nuclear factor-*kappa* B. All statins inhibit this vital step in our immune system's ability to defend us from alien forces. Whether by being the recipient of a donor kidney or under attack by bacteria or viruses, our immune system has evolved a defensive strategy in which inflammation, triggered by nuclear factor-*kappa* B (NF-kB), plays a vital role. Such stimulants to inflammation include the foreign sclerotic and thrombotic changes in our arteries from arterial wall damage. Statin drugs are now known to suppress this nuclear factor-*kappa* B response and thereby open a veritable Pandora's box of unpredictable consequences. [7]

So we have then several different mechanisms of action of the statin class of drugs. The first is cholesterol reduction, a task statins accomplish with great effectiveness in most people. Unfortunately we are now learning that this cholesterol manipulation is irrelevant to atherosclerosis and increased cardiovascular risk. The second action of statins is to inhibit NF-kB and this appears to be the secret to their effectiveness in cardiovascular risk reduction. The third action of statins is a consequence of this NK-kB inhibition, that of altering the effectiveness of our immuno-defense system. [8,9,10,11] The fourth is that of ubiquinone inhibition with its extraordinary consequences relevant to energy production [12,13,14,15] and cell wall integrity [16] and the fifth is dolichol inhibition with its own broad range of potential behavioral manifestations. This sobering information as to the full scope of all statin drugs' potential side effects is completely new to most practicing physicians, who are still trying to cope with the somewhat better understood reality of muscle pain and hepatic inflammation.

Mention must also be given to Red Yeast Rice. This substance has been around for over 3,000 years and contains Mother Nature's purely natural statin, lovastatin (marketed as a pharmaceutical by Merck as Mevacor) derived by the fermentation of rice. As to its potency, there have been many cases of myopathy associated with its use and at least one case of rhabdomyolysis.

One of the more tragic case reports from our unfortunate statin past comes from Steve Sparks,[17] a well-known statin activist. He reports that his father prided himself on doing whatever he could to stay healthy. At the time of being prescribed Baycol, this octogenarian was totally self-supportive, very active in church activities and walked up to 4 miles a day.

He was prescribed Baycol at 0.8 mg on 6 December 2000 for mildly elevated cholesterol and had no other significant medical problems. Within 24 days, he was hospitalized with complete renal failure and a CPK of 150,000. He died on 24th January, 2001. In August 2001, Steve Sparks began his current role as statin drug activist, determined that what had happened to his father should never again happen to any patient.

Despite the belated withdrawal of Baycol, rhabdomyolysis deaths still occur because all currently used statin drugs share the ubiquinone depleting side effect of Baycol, although to a lesser degree. Also relevant are the growing number of reports in the literature of biopsy proven myositis in many patients having muscle soreness unheralded by muscle enzyme elevations telling us that despite reassurances of the drug industry and industry sponsored research, prescribing physicians would be wise to be cautious. The continuing problem of rhabdomyolysis due to statin drugs other than Baycol is best exemplified by the following case report on file both with the FDA's MedWatch and in Dr. Beatrice Golomb's statin study at the University of California San Diego, College of Medicine.[18]

The CEO of a large company began to take Lipitor in 1998 at the time of an emergency angioplasty. His recovery and subsequent course was unremarkable until two things happened to make this 54-year old man both the luckiest and unluckiest man to come to our attention. Generalized muscle pain ushered in his bad luck and the diagnosis was severe rhabdomyolysis manifested by extensive muscle cell breakdown, rising muscle enzyme levels and profound secondary blockage of the kidney tubules by damaged muscle cell debris. Associated with this condition was the loss of respiratory control during sleep and the loss of his ability to express or understand ideas. A physical work-up revealed the usual findings associated with severe rhabdomyolysis muscle cell breakdown but it also included the somewhat surprising presence of a profound loss of short-term memory. Several memory glitches had occurred during the preceding year but he had passed them off as due to lack of concentration. His good luck has been the resourcefulness and support of his wife and family.

He barely survived the rhabdomyolysis and still suffers from pain and weakness. According to his wife, his doctors concur that the damage was somehow caused by Lipitor, a likelihood supported by the failure of extensive testing to show the presence of tumors, stroke or even Alzheimer's. His Lipitor was stopped on 19th January, 2002.

The most alarming episode of this man's transient global amnesia occurred in April of 2002, three months after Lipitor was discontinued. He experienced a 'flashback' reaction comparable to the one that sometimes occurs months after a drug overdose. On 4th April, 2002, as his wife left for work, he volunteered to go to the local store for groceries and, after noting the progressive 'greening' of their swimming pool, added he would pick up some chlorine as well. He did the grocery shopping with the aid of his new hand-held device and several cell-phone calls to his wife about dinner items for the coming weekend. He then went to The Home Depot® to pick up the chlorine and a few other small hardware items. When he parked the car in The Home Depot parking lot he decided to transfer his frozen foods to the trunk before going inside. When he opened the trunk the chlorine and the other items he was planning to buy were sitting there in a Home Depot logo shopping bag. The experience greatly upset him, since he had absolutely no recall of going into Home Depot and buying the items. To add to his befuddlement, when his wife arrived home that evening and checked the receipts, they discovered that the Home Depot chlorine purchase had been made the previous day. No one had been home the previous day when he took out his classic convertible, drove to the store, and then returned home with absolutely no recollection. He was devastated.

When the reality of his memory impairment became clear, other unusual 'memory' lapses were recalled. One of these odd events had occurred almost a year before stopping Lipitor when, while on an errand, he suddenly realized that he was inexplicably heading north on the freeway far away from, and in the wrong direction, for anything he had intended to do. This episode bothered him but he passed it off as preoccupation.

Another odd event had occurred on 27th December, 2001 while they were at their lakeshore camp a few weeks before his life threatening rhabdomyolysis occurred. He had left the house at approximately 4:30 am to do some shore fishing, returning at approximately 8:30 am. When asked if he went fishing he could not recall and was clearly flustered, embarrassed and thoroughly upset over his inability to remember. His wife adds that he must have gone fishing since there is nothing else to do for 40 miles in either direction.

His wife then recalled on 2nd January, 2002, while he was still on Lipitor, he had called her on his cell phone when she was on her way to work. He wanted to know why he was in The Home Depot parking lot. He was not sure why he was there and was flustered, embarrassed and upset not to know. She also recalled that in November and December of 2001 he started some woodworking projects to be used for gifts. After the projects were completed, he would still go into the garage and find wood components already cut, proof that he had restarted the project several times, evidentially forgetting that he had already completed them.

She recorded additional post-Lipitor observations and realized an episode of aberrant behavior occurred on 22 Mar 2002 that fit the TGA profile. Her upset husband had called her at work, from their home, and commented that it had been a bad day. He started out in the morning to go to the office and then to the bank and had placed the banking items on the seat of his car. When he arrived back at home he realized that they were still on the seat so he took the car out again to go to the bank. He set out on the freeway and forgot where he was going. He recalled that when he suddenly looked down and discovered that he was nearly out of gas, he pulled off the freeway and filled the tank. However, at that point he had no idea why he had even been on the freeway or where he was going. It frightened him so much that he went straight home and determined not to leave the house again that day. When told about this, his daughter commented she had seen him on the road and waved at him. He had looked right at her face while she was waving but had not responded. He had no memory of seeing her or her very distinctive car and, since his car was equally distinctive, the chance of either of them making a mistake is very small.

Since 4th April, 2002, no further transient global amnesia-like episodes have been noted. This formerly successful CEO became cognitively impaired and unable to work, testing below the 1st percentile for short-term memory and cognition. Three years of cognitive rehabilitation therapy resulted in a clinical evaluation that stated he could not retain more than a five word sentence long enough to process it and respond. "What do you want for dinner?" at six words, was beyond his capabilities. He was told that his motivation and dedication were such that he was performing to the limits of his capability, but that unless or until regrowth of the damaged nerve tissue occurred, no further capability could be developed.

Now, off Lipitor for a decade—two and a half times the duration of Lipitor exposure—the extreme pain from the peripheral neuropathy has lessened in intensity, indicating nerve tissue regrowth. A correspondingly slow improvement in the ability to form short-term memory has this former CEO currently functioning at approximately 85% of his pre-Lipitor abilities. However, ten years of his life are unrecoverable, due to the inability to form memories during that decade. He must rely on photographs to know of important life events during that period, such as participating in his daughter's wedding.

The Lipitor-induced mitochondrial and neuromuscular damage persists, along with impaired ATP generation. Chronic gout is a problem, as any mild activity beyond 20 minutes results in cell death, which the body halts by releasing uric acid. A few years ago he was diagnosed with diabetes, now known to be consistent with mitochondrial damage, as the legacy of Lipitor damage continues.

Of special interest is the fact that three uneventful years passed before this CEO's Lipitor-associated problems surfaced in the form of his first "memory lapse," and another year was to pass before the dreaded complication of rhabdomyolysis began. This is a sobering observation for those who would seek comfort from the fact that they have been taking a statin drug for a year with no problem. The relationship of this person's short-term memory loss to the rhabdomyolysis remains to be determined. One would surmise that permanent damage to the memory apparatus must have occurred, particularly to the hippocampal area, yet neurologic studies have failed to demonstrate the lesion—an enigma, it would seem.

The statin drugs are in widespread use today and the trend to promote their use even more broadly seems inevitable at present, particularly when one considers the proliferating direct-to-consumer advertising exposure in the U.S. via TV, print, radio and online. One doctor, extremely skeptical that cognitive side effects could be associated with statin drug use, claimed that the only problem with statins lies in the fact that they are not getting to everyone who needs them.

Currently most practicing physicians feel that statins are the best drugs available for high-risk stroke and heart attack patients and are clearly to be recommended when more conservative measures such as diet and exercise are inadequate. There is no doubt that statin drugs substantially reduce cholesterol levels in most people, but there is growing concern among researchers reporting on major clinical trials that cholesterol reduction is not leading to significant reductions in cardiovascular disease mortality.[19,20,21]

Even when statin therapy does seem to increase survival in CHD patients, as reported by Collins, *et al.*, for a large group of diabetics and non-diabetics treated with simvastatin for occlusive arterial disease,[22] one must be wary of the confusing and often misleading use of statistics presented in many randomized controlled trials. For a masterful discussion of the use of statistics to confuse the reader and inflate the true benefit of statin therapy, one need only read Dr. Uffe Ravnskov's book, *The Cholesterol Myths.*[23] (*The Cholesterol Myths is* now out of print but the ideas in it are included and updated in his more recent books "*Fat and Cholesterol Are GOOD for You!*" and "*Ignore the Awkward!*") Additionally, Ravnskov reported on the PROSPER trial published in *The Lancet*, that statin therapy increased the incidence of cancer deaths, completely offsetting the slight decrease in deaths from cardiovascular disease and further complicating interpretation of reported benefits from statin therapy. Most researchers feel this increased number of cancer deaths is based on compromise of the immunodefense system due to NF-kB inhibition.

This observation of increased cancer deaths associated with statin drug use and forecast of more to come was stressed by Paul Rosch, MD in his Weston A. Price Foundation review presentation of May 2003[24]. Support for his concern is evident in the Japan Lipid Intervention Trial observation[25] of excess deaths from malignancy in their so called statin 'hyper-responders,' that sub-group of patients whose total serum cholesterols plummeted to less than 160 mg % during the study period. Of the 12 cancer deaths reported, four were from gastric cancer and 2 were from lung cancer. This heightened cancer risk almost certainly is based on loss of immunoresistance secondary to inhibition of NF-kB, mentioned earlier in this chapter, although other factors may play a role.

Because of this growing specter of doubt about the effectiveness of cholesterol reduction on cardiovascular disease and the risks inherent in statin drug use, there is very real concern about the escalating use of these drugs for primary prevention. Despite a diligent search of the literature, one can find remarkably little support for broader use of the statins for cholesterol reduction.

Moderate hypercholesterolemics—with or without diabetes, obesity, smoking history, hypertension or a family history of the disease—who are now being placed on statin drugs because "everyone knows they are effective and safe," may be better treated by alternative means or by dramatically lowered statin doses.

The physiological implications of these drugs are profound when based on just what is actually known at this time, but when one adds the reality of the present shallow grasp of physiology at the intracellular and molecular level, there is justification for the question, "Do we really know what we are doing?"

So the mechanism of action of the statin class of drugs is far from simple inhibition of cholesterol bio-synthesis. In reality the statin drugs have now been proven to have five distinct faces and even more are likely to be found as research continues. The first face of statins is that of cholesterol reduction. This is a task they do with great efficiency. Lipitor, Zocor (and its offspring Vytorin) take pride in causing up to 40% reduction of total serum cholesterol in many people.

Crestor goes much further with respect to inhibition of cholesterol biosynthesis, claiming as much as a 52 % reduction in many people. But now the results of long-term studies are revealing some remarkable truths. Cholesterol, our nemesis for the past four decades in the fight against cardiovascular disease, has now achieved a position in causality remarkably close to irrelevant. Inflammation is the cause of heightened cardiovascular risk, many researchers are now telling us.

Cholesterol is innocent in its physiologically natural form. Cholesterol is drawn passively into the atherosclerotic plaque by "misguided" LDL. Even our "misguided" LDL may not be LDL at all but a structurally similar substance, known as lipoprotein (a), having a radically different physiological effect. Natural cholesterol is not the cause of the infamous atherosclerotic plaques.

We now have evidence that atherosclerosis is the result of inflammatory factors such as homocysteine, secondary to genetic or acquired deficiencies of vitamin B6, B12 and folic acid. Homocysteine has been shown to be a major player in atherosclerotic change, with coagulation defects, platelet factors and selected anti-oxidant deficiencies responsible for most of the rest. Cholesterol no longer is deserving of even a place in the lineup of usual suspects.

It was only in 2003 that Pfrieger[26] found that the glial cells of the brain provide for brain cholesterol manufacture and are just as effectively inhibited by statins, finally giving an explanation for the bizarre cognitive side effects being reported; the first face of statins' pleiotropic effects. Now we had a mechanism for amnesia, confusion, disorientation, forgetfulness and aggravation of pre-existing senility—the lack of sufficient bioavailability of cholesterol for proper neuronal function. And we must heed particularly the findings of Muldoon[27] that one can document cognitive deterioration in 100% of statin users with the right type of testing.

Now we know the second face of statin drugs, the effective face, the face that no doubt has prevented many cases of heart attacks and strokes. No one seriously argues the positive effects of this happy face but it is anti-inflammatory, not cholesterol lowering. It is a face only recently recognized as the results of long-term studies have been analyzed. Whether your cholesterol goes up, down or remains unchanged, statin drugs work by a means independent of cholesterol reduction. This factor is nuclear factor-*kappa* B, a transcriptase common to our entire immunodefense system.

The pharmaceutical industry has been shocked by this revelation but quick to acknowledge and adapt to the change for now statins are being promoted for organ transplant recipients and as adjunctive therapy in the treatment of auto-immune diseases. Why? Because they work! These results are sobering, indeed, for statin drugs can work in this capacity only at the risk of causing mischief elsewhere.

The third face of statin drug effect is this same nuclear factor-*kappa* B and its effect on the remainder of the immune system. What about cancer and infectious disease? We have had millions of years to work out our defense systems against widely diverse challenges and NF-kB is key to all of them.

Whether by being the recipient of a donor kidney or under attack by bacteria or viruses, or having a mutation induced by radiation in the environment, our immune system has evolved a defensive strategy in which suppression of inflammation, triggered by nuclear factor-*kappa* B, plays a vital role. The ability of statin drugs to suppress this nuclear factor-*kappa* B response is potentially to confound the inner workings of our entire immunodefense system.

Ubiquinone deficiency is the fourth face of statins and the one responsible for the most severe side effects. Statin drugs, while curtailing cholesterol, must inevitably inhibit the production of other vital intermediary products that originate further down the metabolic pathway beyond the statin blockade. The pharmaceutical industry has long been attempting to develop a means by which interference with cholesterol production might be achieved beyond the point where these vital intermediary products originate but up to now have failed. The inevitability of significant, serious and even lethal side effects has been knowingly accepted. Ubiquinone levels plummet when statins are initiated.

Such side effects as congestive heart failure and chronic fatigue reflect ubiquinone's important role in energy production. Hepatitis, myopathy, rhabdomyolysis and peripheral neuropathy reflect ubiquinone's role in cell wall integrity and stability. Ubiquinone's role in the prevention of somatic mitochondrial mutations is also of critical importance and introduces a vast area of concern.

The fifth face of statin drug effect has to do with dolichol availability. Like the ubiquinones, this class of compounds is inevitably collaterally damaged with statin drug use, for it branches off the same biosynthetic tree. Dolichols are vital to the intricate process of neuropeptide formation.

Neuropeptides are biochemicals that regulate almost all life processes on a cellular level, thereby linking all body systems. Although produced primarily in the brain, every cell in the body produces and exchanges neuropeptides. Called messenger molecules, they send chemical messages in the form of linked peptides from the brain to receptor sites on cell membranes throughout the body. Every thought, sensation and emotion we have ever felt has been dependent upon the makeup of these peptide linkages and, surprisingly, they do not simply convey. These peptide clusters are the thought, sensation or emotion in a process we are only just beginning to understand.

We now strongly suspect disruption of this system by statins is behind reports of depression, irritability, hostility, aggressiveness, road rage type behavior, accident and addiction proneness and reports of suicides soon after statin drugs are started.

When confronted by the reality that one's statin is causing intolerable, even dangerous, side effects the question of alternatives or stopping one's statin inevitably arises. A frequent course of action is to try another statin but only rarely does this resolve the problem for all statins are HMG Co-A reductase inhibitors and as such work only in one way —to inhibit the reductase step on the mevalonate pathway of cholesterol biosynthesis. So if you are experiencing muscle pain, short term memory loss, unusual tiredness or depression with your new statin and change to another statin seems futile, what then?

For one who is experiencing the sudden onset of myopathy with rapid progression the answer is obvious; the offending statin is stopped immediately. But for most symptoms, time is not critical and the patient has a choice. Logically, people might ask, "How should I stop my statin, cold turkey, gradual or what?" The problem I see is that increasingly I am seeing reports saying, "I have heard of the side effects of statins from the media (or read about it while internet browsing) and my symptoms were the same. I have stopped my statin and wonder what I should do about my high cholesterol?"

To understand my response, you must understand statins' vital role in reduction of cardiovascular disease risk. Cholesterol has nothing to do with this. Statins' impressive benefits are due solely to their anti-inflammatory action; their powerful ability to inhibit nuclear factor-*kappa* B. This substance is vital to our immune system's function of triggering an inflammatory response to disease. As I mentioned earlier in this book, statins work their magic of lowering cardiovascular disease risk not by cholesterol reduction but by their inherent anti-inflammatory action.

Monocyte adhesion, macrophage recruitment, smooth muscle migration and platelet activation are all parts of the body's defensive inflammatory response, even if such inflammation occurs within the walls of our blood vessels as part of the process of atherosclerosis. Platelet activation is essential to this response to help seal off the disease regardless of its cause. Statins' inhibition of NF-kB reduces the likelihood of thrombosis within our blood vessels during this inflammatory assault, hence its undeniable record in reducing the degree of atherosclerosis and cardiovascular risk. You might recall that aspirin has a similar but far less aggressive effect on platelet function.

Now let us assume you have been on a statin for a few months or years during which time it has provided inhibition of inflammatory activity within your blood vessels. That's good. But then you experience memory loss or severe myopathy and, in consultation with your doctor, must come off statins. When this is done, there is a return of normal platelet activation (stickiness) in most people but some recent studies have shown there will be an overshoot of platelet stickiness, peaking in the second week after stopping the statin. The result is a small but significant tendency for strokes and infarctions to occur during that time. The obvious solution is a gradual tapering off of statins, not abrupt cessation.

My strong belief, then, is that a statin user who, with the approval of his/her doctor, has made the decision to stop his or her statin must do so gradually over at least a two week period. Pill cutters are invaluable for this process. For example, someone on 40mg will cut to 20 for a few days, then 10 for a few days, then 5 and 2.5mg. In this manner any peaking of platelet stickiness will be avoided. I might add that buffered aspirin 81mg during this tapering off phase will be helpful and will also be an important part of an alternative treatment plan of omega-3, CoQ10 and vitamins B6, B12 and folic acid as discussed in the *anti-inflammatory alternatives to statins* chapter.

How strange it is that a class of drugs developed solely for the purpose of interfering with the biosynthesis of cholesterol has now been shown to reduce cardiovascular risk by a novel and unsuspected anti-inflammatory role completely unrelated to cholesterol manipulation. We now have a nation of patients and doctors convinced that cholesterol is public health enemy number one, for none of this recent truth has yet significantly penetrated the hallowed halls of health care delivery. A patient's first question when told their mental aberration or severe muscle pain is most likely a side effect of their statin will often say, "But what can I do about my cholesterol?"

We have a pharmaceutical industry still committed to pushing the charade of cholesterol etiology. Imagine the billions of profit dollars resulting to them from perpetuating the myth of cholesterol? Now, when confronted by the reality of inflammation, they deftly turn their sights towards organ transplant and auto-immune disease.

Perhaps stockholder loyalty explains why Pfizer management knew over a decade ago, during the first human use trial of Lipitor, of the cognitive impact to come when Lipitor was released to the public. Of their 2,503 patients tested with Lipitor, seven experienced transient global amnesia attacks and four others experienced other forms of severe memory disturbances, for a total of 11 cases out of 2,503 test patients. This is a ratio of 4.4 cases of severe cognitive loss to result from every 1000 patients that took the drug. Not one word of warning of this was transmitted to the thousands of physicians who soon would be dispensing the drug. This greatly helps to explain why, when I asked about the Federal Aviation Administration's (FAA's) allowance of statin drug use in commercial airline pilots, one[28] of FAA's leading flight surgeons told me, "I did not know statins could do this."

Today with 30 million patients on statins and using Pfizer's own data, we can expect an astounding 150,000 cases of severe cognitive loss this year alone.

CHAPTER 2
Mevalonate Blockade

The most important side effect of all statin drugs is the inevitable mevalonate blockade they cause. As reductase inhibitors this is predictable. Those taking statins have been drug company guinea pigs for the past 20 years and didn't even know it. Those of you who have been touched by the side effects of statins have every right to be incensed by this reality. Day by day we are learning the true effects of statin drugs on the mevalonate pathway—things the statin drug manufacturers should have known long before they requested FDA approval. But you must remember that back when these drugs were first coming to market, cholesterol was public health enemy number one and these cholesterol inhibitors were high priority. Very few questions were asked by an agency concerned more with rapid approval than picky questions. Anything that would lower cholesterol was a friend of man, no questions asked. Obviously the research scientists knew they were in uncharted water and quite possibly they made their questions and anxieties known to management but in this cost plus effectiveness sparring that took place in the back rooms, research clearly lost to management pressure. Billions of dollars were at stake.

I am not going to tell you these research scientists did not know what was going to happen. Of course they knew the importance of the mevalonate pathway. Of course they knew that blocking this pathway at its very origin was bound to have serious complications. This was their job, their training and their life but they were over-ridden. Billions of dollars create a great deal of pressure, sweetened only by the presumption that if you lower cholesterol 1% you would add 2 years to life. How many times did I hear that in the days of the Framingham study? The anti-cholesterol bandwagon needed the statins badly and whatever safeguards we had, proved to be very flexible. One might say the almighty noise of the bandwagon drowned out the voices of caution and reason. Only in the past decade did the noise of the bandwagon diminish sufficiently to let truths begin to emerge.

The first thing that happened, of course, was the introduction of unnaturally low cholesterol in millions of people. After all that was the purpose of these new statins. Why the drug company and the FDA and the medical community thought these alien values were good for us is very difficult to understand. After all, cholesterol blood levels ranging from 180 to 300 had been around a long time. Then, as if 170 mg % of LDL cholesterol was not low enough, they lowered the standard to capture more "sick" people needful of treatment. For a time the desirable level then became 140, then 120, now 100 and in special cases 70 mg%. Obviously if they lowered their desirable cholesterol level sufficiently the entire population of the world would have this new disease. The term medical mafia comes to mind as in my mind I see HMO administrators and pharmaceutical CEOs rub their palms in glee while dreaming of truly scandalous profits to come. And all this time new research was demonstrating unusual associations of low cholesterol with such things as premature birth, small birth weight, congenital anomalies, poverty, lower intelligence and sociopathic behavior.

Then the consequences of CoQ10 inhibition gradually leaked out. A major part of the mevalonate pathway is directed at CoQ10 synthesis (see the Mevalonate Pathway figure on the back cover). As a consequence, CoQ10 plummets after statins are started and one person after another was reporting muscle damage, rhabdomyolysis, neuropathy, congestive heart failure, weakness and serious fatigue all related one way or another to lack of CoQ10. CoQ10 supplementation when started was usually at the patient's insistence, not the doctor's.

Then, in 2001 we learned of Frank Pfreiger's[1] astounding revelation of the importance of cholesterol to brain function. The brain's synapses cannot function without sufficient cholesterol and since the LDL/cholesterol molecule is much too large to pass the blood-brain barrier, nature has devised an alternative means of manufacture; the housekeeping cells of the brain, known as glial cells. We have been eons evolving this special mechanism for brain cholesterol supply and the biochemists at Big Pharma had no clue as to what they had done. Of course, these glial cells were extremely sensitive to statins' touch and finally in 2003 we had an explanation for the amnesia, forgetfulness, confusion and disorientation.

Meanwhile the statins had been on the market for 15 years and these almost inevitable cognitive side effects were being overlooked by thousands of physicians completely unaware about the cognitive impairment potential of the statins. "You're getting older," or, "Perhaps a touch of Alzheimer's?" was the prevailing excuse for this terrible oversight. And the hundreds of cases of elderly patients passing in dementia shortly after statins were started "For their health" are best left buried.

And what was the reaction of Big Pharma to this news of their gross culpability in the cognitive damage to millions of Americans? Dead silence! Their reaction was to say nothing and do nothing. Their damage control people knew that few doctors read the science journals anyhow and it would be much better for marketing and sales to say no more about it. The entire thing would blow over in a few weeks and that is exactly what happened. Had management decided to apologize for this tragic oversight, the multibillion dollar statin drug industry would have disappeared overnight. As it turned out, today you have to look hard to find a doctor who knows of statins' effect on memory.

Then, only a few years ago, did we learn of the close association of statin therapy with aggression[2], hostility, irritability, homicidal ideation, depression and suicides and only then did we know that the likely mechanism of action was our dolichols, which bear the entire responsibility for overseeing our neuropeptide synthesis function. Every thought, every sensation and every emotion you have ever had originates with the synthesis of a specific neuropeptide strand. Dolichols are collaterally damaged by statins, just like

CoQ10. By now, statins had been on the market for 18 years and patient claims of bizarre thoughts and actions during this time had been swept under the carpet as emotional by the unsuspecting physicians and referred to psychiatry.

The reason for this inevitable evolution of statin drug side effects was the mevalonate pathway. In their focus on cholesterol the drug industry had effectively blocked this entire pathway, shared by CoQ10 synthesis, dolichol synthesis, normal phosphorylation, selenoprotein synthesis and other vital functions. To get at the cholesterol branch of the mevalonate tree they had girded the entire tree at its origin. Anyone who has ever raised a tree will tell you, you can't do that! Once you gird the trunk of the tree, all branches are affected. That is just as predictable as night following day.

And there is more, much more. On the basis of my years of research I could talk selenoprotein inhibition, tau protein synthesis and other new pathways of a statin drug's broad reach but I have made my point. Those that have been on statins have all been guinea pigs. Welcome to the club!

But there is one more observation that I saved for the end—*la pièce de résistance*. The fact is that now we have learned that cholesterol is irrelevant to the atherosclerotic process.[3,4] Inflammation is the cause and statins work because they are powerful suppressors of inflammation[5]. Cholesterol, the reason the statins were developed in the first place, is probably our closest biochemical friend. Research scientists were completely ignorant of this anti-inflammatory aspect of statin drugs. This was just serendipity. Atherosclerosis benefits by this effect but the benefit is unacceptable at the cost of the mevalonate pathway.

In reality one of the best ways to overcome this problem is to have physicians open their dusty textbooks of biochemistry and check first the mevalonate pathway of cholesterol synthesis and then review the oxidation phosphorylation dependence upon CoQ10. I can hear the groans of intellectual awakening now and the murmurs of, "I didn't know statins could do that."

CHAPTER 3
Statins and Brain Cholesterol

Pfreiger's announcement on 9 November 2001 about the discovery of the identity of the elusive synaptogenic factor responsible for the development of synapses, the highly specialized contact sites between adjacent neurons in the brain[1], deserves to be cited again in the context of cholesterol's vast importance to our bodies. Not surprisingly to specialists in the field, the synaptogenic factor was shown to be the notorious substance cholesterol!

The so-called glial cells, the non-nervous or supporting tissue of the brain and spinal cord long suspected of providing certain housekeeping functions, were shown to produce their own supply of cholesterol for the specific purpose of providing nerve cells with this vital synaptic component. As many of you may know, the neuronal synapse of the nervous system is the basis of neurotransmission connecting the brain with the rest of the body. The brain cannot tap the cholesterol supply in the blood because the lipoproteins that carry cholesterol—both LDL and HDL—in the blood are too large to pass the blood-brain barrier[2]. The brain must depend upon its own cholesterol synthesis, which the glial cells provide.

This should be sobering news for those in the pharmaceutical industry developing drugs which interfere with cholesterol synthesis, and that is exactly the mechanism of action of all statins. One wonders how anyone knowing the mechanism of brain cholesterol synthesis can seriously challenge the reality of cognitive side effects from statin drug use. The only surprise is that there are not more reported cases of memory impairment, amnesia, confusion and disorientation.

After years of reader queries about statin drugs use, I have learned that very few people, many prescribing physicians included, know of the full range of side effects of the statin class of drugs.

I suppose my first rude awakening on the prevalence of this lack of knowledge among physicians about the drugs they prescribe was during my own personal experience with transient global amnesia bouts after taking Lipitor. On both occasions, dozens of physicians with whom I came in contact said, "Lipitor doesn't do that."

Dozens of pharmacists during that same time period said the same thing, "Statins don't do that." Now that a statin study has reported nearly one thousand cases of statin associated transient global amnesia, physicians are reluctantly accepting the reality of amnesia, confusion, disorientation, extreme forgetfulness and aggravation of pre-existing senility but many still do not know it exists.

The following personal account has now been replayed hundreds of times in emergency rooms throughout the world as statin users are seen for their amnesias. Mine was one of the first statin associated transient global amnesia (TGA) cases reported to the UCSD statin study.

My personal introduction to the incredible world of TGA occurred six weeks after Lipitor was started during my annual astronaut physical at Johnson Space Center. My cholesterol had been trending upward for several years and all was well until six weeks later when my wife found me aimlessly walking about the yard after I returned from my usual walk in the woods. I did not recognize her, reluctantly accepted cookies and milk and refused to go into my now unfamiliar home. I "awoke" six hours later in the office of the examining neurologist with the diagnosis of transient global amnesia, cause unknown. My MRI several days later was normal. Since Lipitor was the only new medicine I was on, the doctor in me made me suspect a possible side effect of this drug and, despite the protestations of the examining doctors that statin drugs did not do this, I stopped my Lipitor.

The year passed uneventfully and soon it was time for my next astronaut physical. NASA doctors joined the chorus I had come to expect from physicians and pharmacists during the preceding year, that statin drugs did not do this and at their bidding I reluctantly restarted Lipitor at one-half the previous dose. Six weeks later I again descended into the black pit of amnesia, this time for twelve hours and with a retrograde loss of memory back to my high school days. During that terrible interval, when my entire adult life had been eradicated, I had no awareness of my marriage and children, my medical school days, my ten adventure-filled years as a USAF flight surgeon or my selection as NASA scientist astronaut. All had vanished from my mind as completely as if they had never happened. Fortunately, and typically for this obscure condition, my memory returned spontaneously and again I drove home listening to my wife's amazing tale of how my day (and hers) had gone.

The medical literature is now replete with reports of statin associated amnesias and other evidence of mental dysfunction and still many of our prescribing physicians remain unaware of statins' special cognitive impairment tendency. Their patient's rapid descent into dementia after a statin is started is much too often written off by their doctor as senile brain changes or beginning Alzheimer's when the real culprit is their statin drug.

Readers will be interested to know of Muldoon's reports in the medical literature documenting cognitive impairment in 100% of statin users if sufficiently sensitive testing is done.[3]

Transient global amnesia is the sudden inability to formulate new memory, known as anterograde amnesia, combined with varying degrees of retrograde memory loss, sometimes for decades into the past.[4] Until recently, the most common trigger events for these abrupt and completely unheralded amnesia cases have been sudden vigorous exercise, sexual activity, emotional crises, cold water immersion, trauma—at times quite subtle—and cerebral angiography. In the past years a new trigger agent has been added; the use of the stronger statin drugs such as Lipitor, Zocor (and its derivative, Vytorin) Mevacor and Crestor.

Transient global amnesia is but the tip of the iceberg of the many other forms of statin associated memory lapses that are reported from distraught patients.[5] Far more common are symptoms of disorientation, confusion, unusual forgetfulness or increasing senility symptoms. These lesser forms of memory impairment can be easily missed in many individuals because, to a certain degree, that is the nature of us all.

Explanation for statin drugs' effect on our cognition first came on 9th November, 2001 when Dr. Pfreiger of the Max Planck Society for the Advancement of Science announced that without abundant supplies of cholesterol, normal synaptic function cannot take place. Synapses are the connections between our neurons. Our neurons are what we are. We are not precise creatures and most of us know it. Few will deny the tendency of our minds for occasional very sketchy recall. Constant vigilance is necessary to keep us from "wandering."

Knowing the inevitable effect of statins on cholesterol availability to our brains, I sadly shake my head when I read reports where thousands of people were placed on high doses of statins for a special study and their supervising physicians report no significant side effects. In my world, experiencing a constant stream of statin adverse reports, "no significant side effects" from that dose of statins is simply not possible.

Charged by nature with the specific task of synthesizing cholesterol for brain function, the glial cells in our brains are just as sensitive to the effect of statins as any other cell in our bodies. The pharmaceutical industry must have quivered a bit on that surprising news from Pfrieger in 2001 but you would never have known it from their response.

So now we have a thoroughly documented mechanism of action for the hundreds of TGA's and other forms of cognitive dysfunction associated with (and possibly even inevitable with) the use of statins. Knowing of this, how is it possible for any responsible physician to say, "Statins don't do this?"

CHAPTER 4
Statins and CoQ10

We must next consider the impaired production of our vital ubiquinone coenzyme, a collaterally damaged area of great concern since the biochemical ramifications are both broad and profound. Ubiquinone is arguably our most important essential nutrient.[1] Its role in energy production is to make possible the transfer of electrons from one protein complex to another within the inner membrane of the mitochondria to its ultimate recipient, adenosine triphosphate (ATP). The adult human body pool of this substance has been reported to be 2 grams and requires replacement of about 0.5 grams per day.[2] This must be supplied by endogenous synthesis or dietary intake. Synthesis decreases progressively in humans above age 21 and the average ubiquinone content of the western diet is less than 5 mg/day.

Thus, ubiquinone supplementation appears to be the only way for older people to obtain their daily need of this important nutrient. Tens of millions of people will be taking statins this year in the United States alone. Most of these people will be over 50 years of age. Few of them will be on supplemental ubiquinone. Simple logic dictates that the statin drug impact on ubiquinone availability and mitochondrial energy production will be profound!

Because of the extremely high energy demands of the heart, this organ is usually the first to feel statin-associated CoQ10 depletion as cardiomyopathy and congestive heart failure. The importance of mitochondrial function in meeting the energy needs of the heart has been emphasized recently because of the increasing tendency for congestive heart failure (CHF) in statin drug users.[3] Peter Langsjoen MD, well-known cardiologist, has published a series of excellent articles on this subject[4] and reviewed the prevalence of statin associated CHF in many controlled studies, reporting on the prompt response of CHF to supplemental ubiquinone or reductions in statin dosage.

Perhaps it should be added here that the heart as an organ is just another striated muscle, presumably subject to the same statin-related pathology as the rhabdomyolysis of muscles in general. But the cardiomyopathy of congestive heart failure seems based primarily in the depletion of energy reserves at the mitochondrial level. However, both myopathy in general and cardiomyopathy relate strongly to statin drug depletion of coenzyme Q10 reserves.

Ubiquinone in a slightly altered form known as ubiquinol is found in all membranes where it has a vital function in maintaining membrane integrity. Liver inflammation, with breakdown of liver cells releasing their enzymes into the bloodstream and thereby serving as a marker of statin damage, is likely due, at least in part, to loss of cell wall integrity. Breakdown of cell walls secondary to excessive ubiquinol inhibition by statin drug use is suspected to be involved in both the neuropathy and myopathy case reports now flooding the literature. Myopathy, if sufficiently severe, may lead to rhabdomyolysis, a condition wherein muscle cell walls break down and release myoglobin causing secondary blockage of kidney tubules. Baycol was removed from the market primarily on the basis of excessive tendency for muscle cell damage and breakdown. Unfortunately, many deaths resulted before this corrective action was taken. And have rhabdomyolysis deaths now disappeared? The answer is no, for it is inherent in all statins. Patients still die from this statin side effect on muscles but at lower rates, less irritating to FDA's eyes perhaps, but still grossly irritating to mine in view of cholesterol's irrelevancy in cardiovascular disease risk.

Dr. David Gaist[5] in a study of 116 patients reported a 16 times greater risk of polyneuropathy among long term statin drug users. This new and very serious side effect of statins should be of special concern to diabetics, many of whom have been prescribed statins because of their high-risk status. All doctors know that a very common outcome of long standing diabetes is peripheral neuropathy. To prescribe statins with their established record of neuropathy to these patients because of their special predisposition to heart attack and stroke is a serious decision, a delicate balance of judgment that should be undertaken only after painful soul-searching on the part of the doctor. This is the so-called art of medicine—making the right choice of medicines when considering more than one variable.

And thousands have reported muscle aches and pains from myopathy, the most commonly reported side effect of statin drug use. Some of these have negative tests for the enzyme CPK[6], representing a growing sub-group of statin damage cases. Such cases presumably represent a "contained" inflammatory response, wherein muscle cell wall integrity is maintained despite the intracellular turmoil. Many statin users report using muscle discomfort as an indicator of statin dosage and will adjust their statin dose up or down depending on presence or absence of muscle pain. One might call this fool-hardy stunt the equivalent of "dancing with the devil" for they are always right on the edge of serious muscle damage in their efforts to maintain "health."

Ubiquinone is also vital to the formation of elastin and collagen. Tendon and ligament inflammation and rupture have frequently been reported by statin drug users and it is likely that the mechanism of this predisposition to damage is related to some yet unknown compromise of ubiquinone's role in connective tissue formation. I have received hundreds of reports reflecting unusual susceptibility of ligaments and tendons to damage while on statin drugs.

There is still another thoroughly documented role for ubiquinone, just as important as mitochondrial energy production and cell wall integrity. That is its role within the mitochondria as a powerful anti-oxidant[7], with a free radical quenching ability some 50 times greater than that of vitamin E. Without adequate stores of ubiquinone and lacking the repair mechanisms common to nuclear DNA, irreversible oxidative damage to mitochondria DNA results from buildup of superoxide and hydroxyl radicals. We must remember that our mitochondria are in immediate contact with oxygen, front line warriors, so to speak, in our struggle to obtain life-giving oxygen without sustaining excessive oxidative damage. The inevitable result of excessive free radical accumulation is an increase in the rate of mitochondrial mutations. According to some the cumulative effect of somatic mitochondrial mutations may contribute directly to many chronic myopathies, diabetes and even aging.[8]

Ubiquinone synthesis inhibition secondary to the newer, stronger class of statin drugs is well known to the pharmaceutical industry which has toyed with the idea of recommending that supplemental Coenzyme Q10 be used by patients on statins. Strangely enough the major adverse effect of all statins was sufficiently well known to Merck, the originator of Mevacor, that Merck applied for two patents. The patents were for a combination statin/CoQ10 pill. Under justification for adding CoQ10 to their statin they said "to help prevent the inflammation to come." The patents were granted in 1990 and simply filed away by Merck.

This oversight by Merck laid the groundwork for Dr. Sidney Wolfe's petition of 20 August 2001[10] and Dr. Julian Whitaker's 23 May 2002 petition[11] to the Food and Drug Administration (FDA). Dr. Whitaker's petition called on the commissioner of the FDA to change the package insert on all statin drugs and to issue a "black box" warning to consumers of the need to take coenzyme Q10 (CoQ10) whenever they take a statin drug. The government of Canada requires a warning on all statins that states that these drugs significantly reduce circulating levels of CoQ10.

The following are a few reports from individuals that have written to me dealing primarily with excessive inhibition of Coenzyme Q10:

"I am experiencing many of the side effects listed for Lipitor. I have been taking it for quite some time but the worst symptoms are fairly recent. Would this be possible? I have finally been told I have fibromyalgia, which has similar symptoms and problems. Since I read about the fact that Lipitor can be causing muscle problems even when you have a normal CPK I just yesterday stopped taking it to see if it helps. I have muscle and joint pain, cognitive problems, lack

of attention, restless leg syndrome, irritable bowel syndrome, problems walking because my hips begin to hurt so badly and extreme fatigue."

"I am 45. When I was in my early 30's my blood levels for cholesterol were measured at over 700. It was so high that they had to dilute my blood to get a measurement because at the time the readings they were using only went to 400. My triglycerides levels were ~2000 (if memory serves me correctly). I was put on Mevacor at a fairly high dose and my levels only came down to mid-300's. They increased my dosage to the maximum and it came down to the high 200's (280'ish). Soon after taking this level my muscles petered out and my Doc was puzzled. This was very early on in the history of statins and I was one of the first patients that my Doc had that was taking Mevacor at the higher dose. He did some research and had me back off some and add niacin at 3 grams a day. My blood profile looked great for 10 years - 160 total with a 67 HDL; life was good. About 12 months ago things started going south. My levels started to edge back up. I lost my energy and doing simple tasks gave me very sore muscles. I would wake up in the morning all stiff and there were some days where I would not want to even move. The fatigue became so great that I would have a hard time staying awake while driving the 11 miles to work. On the worst days my entire body would be so sore it reminded me of the day after my first day of skiing for the season - but for no reason! My CPK levels have been measure at 313; high but not alarmingly so. However my (new) Doc has told me to taper off my meds until the CPK levels come back down; he does not care about my cholesterol levels at this point. I have been doing research on the web and have found a lot of info indicating that C-Q10 levels could be the real problem. I have taken 200mg for 2 days and I already am starting to feel better. I am still looking for answers but I feel that I am at last on the correct path."

CHAPTER 5
Statins and Dolichols

Science has amassed so much research knowledge that very little remains simple and straightforward, so one ventures cautiously into the murky complexity of another secondary metabolite potentially compromised by statin drug use, that of the dolichols. The role of dolichols in the manufacture of neuropeptides is an intricate process of cellular activity that has fascinated researchers for years.[1] Neuropeptides are biochemicals that regulate almost all life processes on a cellular level, thereby linking all body systems.[2,3,4,5] Although produced primarily in the brain, every tissue in the body produces and exchanges neuropeptides. Called messenger molecules, they send chemical messages from the brain to receptor sites on cell membranes throughout the body.

Until recently such intercellular information transfer was felt to be the sole province of our classic neurotransmitter chemicals such as serotonin and catecholamines, gate-keepers of our synapses, aided by various hormones carried by our vascular system. Now we have learned that not only do neuropeptides supplement these systems, they provide the vast majority of information transfer. Not only do these protein chains carry information throughout the body, they also mysteriously seem to be the information. They do not simply convey thought, sensation or emotion; these peptide clusters are the thought, sensation or emotion in a process we are only just beginning to understand.

Within each of our cells are minuscule factories of immense complexity. Floating in the cytoplasm is a tubular network of membranes called the endoplasmic reticulum. It is here that peptide units are linked one by one into what amounts to a tiny chain, with the ultimate cellular message of each neuropeptide chain, whether anger or love, dependent on the exact sequence and composition of these links. Imagine, every sensation or emotion one has ever experienced, depending upon the makeup of these short neuropeptide chains, like popcorn on a string, carrying our behavioral destiny. These linked peptides are then packaged into transport vesicles that are shuttled across the cytoplasm to the Golgi apparatus. The operation of the Golgi apparatus, this marvel of complexity, which only recently has begun to reveal its secrets to research scientists, has been likened to that of a post office. Electron microscopy has revealed that its general structure is comparable to a stack of "letters" shaped like hotcakes and bound by a common membrane. It is here in vesicles that proteins are linked with certain sugars, zip-code fashion, and directed to their final destination within and without the cell, and it is here that the dolichols play their unique role. In the absence of sufficient dolichol this delicate process cannot properly take place.

We are now familiar with the blocking action of statins on ubiquinone but few really understand the consequence of dolichol suppression by statin drug use. When I was in medical school, dolichols and neuropeptides were unknown or much too vague a concept to talk about. Few physicians readily comprehend what has been learned in the past few decades without having done detailed study of journals of biochemistry and molecular biology, so few practicing physicians will find this material familiar. Without sufficient dolichols, the intricate process of neuropeptide formation and transport cannot occur. Intracellular chaos can result, as various proteins are not directed to their proper target and are, in effect, dead-lettered. The post office analogy, though childishly simple, comes very close to describing the Golgi apparatus function as we understand it today and the entire process is orchestrated by dolichols.

There is no disputing either statins' inhibition of dolichol synthesis or dolichol's vital role in neuropeptide formation. Since our neuropeptides are involved in so many areas of physiology, possible manifestations of impaired neuropeptide function are protean, suggesting that even the most obscure of patient symptoms may be associated with statin use. Researchers in this field are reporting the frequent association of statin use with such symptoms as hostility, aggressiveness, irritability, homicidal actions, road rage type behavior, exacerbation of alcohol and drug addiction, proneness to depression, suicidal thoughts, failed suicidal attempts and occasional suicide successes.[6] Such behavioral manifestations are felt to be related to dolichol inhibition and altered neuropeptide formation.

The following are just two of the many reports I have received from people who report emotional and behavioral side effects associated with their use of statin drugs:

"My father who is 70 years, about 3 months ago started having pressure on the right side of his head and nervousness - he feels like he is losing his mind - he says it feels like something is crawling inside his legs - he is miserable. His primary care physician says it is depression and increased his Zoloft - that has been 2 weeks ago - and he is no better. He says his mind just won't let him think - and everything seems confusing to him. I tried to talk with the physician about the Lipitor that he has been taking for years - because I saw on the internet that Lipitor could cause problems with patients who were also on Lanoxin (it said it could build up a toxin). The physician won't have it any other way but depression - I just don't see that - my father has never been depressed a day in his life."

My mother has struggled with high cholesterol for many years, specifically with her triglyceride levels. Diet did not alter her levels. I may add that she is an active 66-year who walks 4 miles a day, and is in great physical shape. About 9 months ago, my siblings and I noticed that she did not call us as much, and that when we talked with her by phone or in person, she seemed to not recall past conversations or details. She has gotten worse, where she seems withdrawn from conversations, and uninterested in things that happen around her. This is not all of the time, as sometimes she seems like her old self. She is a recently retired RN who worked for 30 years in the field. She is currently taking Lipitor and Pravachol to control the cholesterol, and has been put on a mild dose of medication to stimulate the brain (unsure of its name, but is used to treat early signs of dementia). I have produced two articles from the Wall Street Journal regarding the statin drugs and the effect on memory for my dad who has taken them to the physician. He was told that they are a top-notch treatment center, which none of us denies, and that statin drugs do not affect the memory. My obvious first thought is to seek another opinion, and to take her off of the statins to see if this makes a difference. If the memory loss is caused by the Lipitor, then we can deal with that, but if it is the beginnings of something more serious, then a different approach to my siblings and I would be in order to take advantage of her now."

CHAPTER 6
Statins and Nuclear Factor-*kappa* B (NF-kB)

Even if the dedicated researchers of the pharmaceutical industry discover a way around the side effect mechanisms already described, even greater hurdles exist from recent evidence that statins work not by cholesterol manipulation but by some basic anti-inflammatory mechanism.

Key to this is a substance known as nuclear factor-*kappa* B. All statins inhibit the synthesis of this vital stuff in our immune system's ability to defend us from alien forces.[1] Whether by being the recipient of a donor kidney or under attack by bacteria or viruses, our immune system has evolved a defensive strategy in which suppression of inflammation, triggered by nuclear factor-*kappa* B, plays a vital role.[2] Such stimulants to inflammation include the foreign by-products of arterial inflammation and damage. Statin drugs are known to suppress this nuclear factor-*kappa* B response and thereby open a completely novel opportunity for unpredictable and potentially disastrous consequences.

At best, HMG Co-A reductase inhibitors are blunt instruments and our immuno-defense system is both delicate and complex. During eons of co-existence of our complex multicellular life forms with competing, simpler unicellular organisms, there have developed many different forms of defensive and offensive strategies, all dealing with the needs of one or the other of these dueling organisms to gain a survival advantage.[3,4,5] We have had millions of years to work out our defense systems against widely diverse challenges and NF-kB is key to all of them. If we thought the complexity of cholesterol manufacture by the body is complex, it is child's play compared to what is involved in anti-infection and immunomodulation. Now, throw in a statin and try to predict the consequences.

NF-kB in its several forms is known to molecular biologists as a transcription factor and my bringing more than a smattering of this complex subject to your attention would risk losing you from terminal boredom, so skim the following very lightly. I warned you this is challenging—how could the history of a 3.5 billion year war be otherwise? NF-kB resides in the cytoplasm of each cell in five different forms known to molecular biologists as family. The offspring of these family members, known as dimers, remain firmly held in check in the cytoplasm by certain inhibitory proteins until a release signal is received, allowing our now activated NF-kB to enter the nucleus of the cell. It is there, in the nucleus, that it completes its mission in life to stimulate genes and manufacture proteins necessary for such diverse tasks as monocyte adhesion, macrophage recruitment, smooth muscle migration and platelet activation, key elements of our defensive inflammatory response.

With so many steps involved, a good strategist could predict many different forms of assault by dedicated viruses, bacteria and other forms of single celled life, for this war is basically that of the monocellular rulers originally dominating life on our planet against us multicellular usurpers. Therefore it should come as no surprise that some of these defenders have managed to gain an advantage over us, their adversary, by inhibiting NF-kB while others succeed by enhancing NF-kB.[6,7,8,9]

Others manage both sides of the coin. E.coli, one of the most common infectious agents, prevents NF-kB from entering the nucleus, thereby enabling this ubiquitous organism freer access to the bladder walls and urethra. Through a similar process of checkmate, another common bacteria, *Salmonella*, inhibits our anti-inflammatory response sufficiently long to allow bacterial colonization of the lining of the gut, giving a decided advantage to "their" side. On the other hand, some *Chlamydia* organisms, warring against the urogenital systems of both men and women, have evolved a distinct advantage by enhancing NF-kB, thereby assuring increased survival of infected cells in our urinary and reproductive systems. On a far more serious note, the very common Epstein-Barr virus causing infectious mononucleosis uses NF-kB inhibition to help destroy our protective "T" cells as part of the common teenage "mono" presentation but when it decides to go on a malignant rampage, triggering nasopharyngeal carcinoma and Burkitt's lymphoma, it does so through sustained NF-kB activation. The list goes on and on with other microorganisms and foreign antigens of all kinds, numbering thousands of variations of these basic themes.

So now let us return to statin drugs and their now well-established effect of inhibition of NF-kB. What does this really mean in our ancient struggle with disease organisms and our immune system's competence? It means that while taking statins we are likely to be far more susceptible to certain common infectious agents but at the same time may be somewhat more resistant to others. In the case of the Epstein Barr virus, perhaps we will see more "mono" but, fortunately, less nasopharyngeal carcinoma and Burkitt's lymphoma. But the reality is that we do not as yet know because this new statin role of NF-kB inhibition has only just been recognized. The potential for increased risk of both infectious disease and malignancy is there, for both depend upon our immune system's competence. Tossing the statin sledgehammer into this system is perhaps quite comparable in effect to the rampages of "a bull in a china shop" and it is far too soon to tell about most malignant changes. The implications of the very recent drug company promotion of statin drugs for organ transplant recipients and as adjunctive therapy in the treatment of auto-immune diseases[10,11] are sobering, indeed, for these drugs can only work in this capacity at the risk of causing mischief elsewhere. One must admire the drug companies' ability for "positive spin" on a very alarming proposition, or is it arrogance? One cannot have the one without the other. The sense of cynicism here is overwhelming to me.

Increased cancer deaths among recipients of statin drugs already are being observed. Ravnskov in his book, *The Cholesterol Myths*, has reported from the PROSPER trial[12] that statin therapy increased the incidence of cancer deaths, completely offsetting the slight decrease in deaths from cardiovascular disease. As Dr. Paul Rosch predicted in his Weston A. Price Foundation presentation of May 2003,[13] the Japan Lipid Intervention trial observed excess deaths from malignancy in their so-called statin "hyper-responder" group.[14] Of the 12 cancer deaths reported in this group, whose cholesterols plummeted deeply with statin use, four were from gastric cancer and two were from lung cancer. Although other factors may have played a role, this heightened cancer risk may well be based on at least partial loss of immunoresistance secondary to NF-kB inhibition.

How strange it is that a class of drugs developed solely for the purpose of interfering with the biosynthesis of cholesterol has now been shown to reduce cardiovascular risk by an anti-inflammatory role completely unrelated to cholesterol manipulation. Generally speaking this should by a welcome observation, for atherosclerosis with all of its consequences is based primarily upon inflammation within the arterial walls. Now, however, any optimism we might have had is thoroughly tempered by the growing realization that statins' effect is based upon interference with our most basic immuno defense system. The potential consequences are frightening.

CHAPTER 7
The Role of Cholesterol in the Body

There is no doubt that the present notoriety of cholesterol has all but obscured its physiological importance and necessity in our bodies. Cholesterol is not only the most common organic molecule in the brain, it is also distributed intimately throughout the entire body. It is an essential constituent of the membrane surrounding every cell. The presence of cholesterol in this fatty double layer of the cell wall adjusts the fluidity and rigidity of this membrane to the proper value for both cell stability and function.

Additionally, cholesterol is the precursor for a whole class of hormones known as the steroid hormones that are absolutely critical for life, as we know it. These hormones determine our sexuality, control the reproductive process, and regulate blood sugar levels and mineral metabolism. This same substance that society has been taught to fear happens to be our sole source for androgen, estrogen and progesterone. Researchers marvel at the remarkable similarity in chemical structure these sex hormones have with each other and with the original cholesterol parent from which they are derived. One might say the glaring family resemblance attests to the mighty power of a methyl group here and a carboxyl group there. The destiny of us all is marvelously controlled by such seemingly minor changes.

This same notorious cholesterol substance is also the parent of a pair of steroid hormones called aldosterone and cortisol.[1] Aldosterone protects the body from excessive loss of sodium and water and is known in scientific circles as a mineralocorticoid. It is absolutely vital for life. Without an adequate supply of aldosterone we would be like an ill-prepared desert traveler destined to die of thirst and dehydration under the glaring rays of a merciless sun as water and salt escape from his body.

Cortisol is known as a glucocorticoid because it helps control blood sugar levels and glucose metabolism, but it also has powerful mineralocorticoid and immune system functions and is fundamentally involved in the biologic response to the stress in our lives.

Both of these vital substances are created in the cortex, the outer shell of the adrenal glands. When the adrenal cortex is destroyed by accident, surgery or disease, death occurs within days unless the patient receives aldosterone and cortisol. Like the sex hormones mentioned above, there can be no aldosterone or cortisol unless an adequate supply of the parent substance, cholesterol, is available. So much of our life is dependent on this remarkable substance.

And where would we be without calcitriol?[2] Another offspring of cholesterol, this remarkable steroid hormone is charged with the responsibility for maintaining the proper level of calcium in our bodies. Like sodium, serum calcium must be maintained by the body within a very narrow range for us to function. Without calcitriol the calcium we ingest would pass through our bowels unclaimed. The calcium in our teeth and bones would diminish rapidly, leading to advanced osteoporosis, skeletal weakness and fractures. Without calcium, nerve transmission to our muscles would fail, resulting in a hyperexcitable state. We have all seen cartoons and movies where a doctor gets an exaggerated knee jerk response while checking a patient's reflexes, a sure sign of low calcium levels. Very low calcium levels result in massive seizures of muscles, incompatible with life, in a condition known as generalized tetany. Such is the power of a simple element like calcium on our bodies if homeostatic levels are violated. Proper levels of serum calcium are also vital for optimum function of our immune systems.

Again, cholesterol is the basis of all these steroid hormones without which life, as we know it, would not be possible. But, by no means is the list of cholesterol's contributions to body function exhausted, for there is another class of cholesterol's steroid offspring without which our metabolic well-being might be in serious jeopardy: the production of bile acids. Secreted by the liver and stored in the gall bladder, bile makes it possible for us to emulsify fats and other nutrients. Without bile, we could not digest and absorb the fats in our diet. In the absence of sufficient bile acids we would all be like those unfortunate souls whose intestinal villi are rudimentary or deficient, which causes them to produce voluminous stools of undigested material while they slowly starve.

The pharmaceutical industry would lead us to believe that rapidly bottoming out our natural cholesterol levels through the use of their highly touted statin drugs is a relatively innocuous process of definite benefit to society. But as we learn more each day of this ubiquitous and unique substance, we must question the veracity of their medical advisors. Cholesterol is perhaps the most important substance in our lives for we could not live without an abundant supply of it. Researchers everywhere are learning how extraordinarily complex and often surprising are the pathways that produce and metabolize cholesterol in our bodies. Admittedly, even after decades of study of this remarkable chemical, we still have much to learn.

Pfreiger's announcement on 9th November, 2001 about the discovery of the identity of the elusive synaptogenic factor responsible for the development of synapses, the highly specialized contact sites between adjacent neurons in the brain, deserves to be cited again in the context of cholesterol's vast importance to our bodies.[3] Neuronal transmission, the very essence of who we are, is absolutely dependent upon abundant cholesterol reserves. The synaptogenic factor was shown to be the notorious substance cholesterol!

The so-called glial cells, the non-nervous or supporting tissue of the brain and spinal cord long suspected of providing certain housekeeping functions, were shown to produce their own supply of cholesterol for the specific purpose of providing nerve cells with this vital synaptic component.

This should be sobering news for those in the pharmaceutical industry developing drugs which interfere with cholesterol synthesis, the mechanism of action of all the statins. One wonders how anyone knowing the mechanism of brain cholesterol synthesis by our glial cells can seriously challenge the reality of cognitive side effects from statin drug use. The only surprise is that there are not more reported cases of memory impairment, amnesia, confusion and disorientation.

This is heady stuff, indeed, for a substance with such bad press. When and if the industry finally vindicates cholesterol, it will not be unlike posthumously elevating Al Capone to knighthood.

This discussion of the biological importance of cholesterol would not be complete without a review of recent research information concerning some of the other more sobering implications of excessively low serum cholesterol concentrations in our bodies.

Despite Muldoon's findings of no increase in suicides, accidents and violence in his cholesterol lowering treatment groups,[5] Golomb reported a significant association between low or lowered cholesterol levels and violence across many types of studies.[6] As principal investigator of the National Institutes of Health funded study at University of California San Diego, College of Medicine, Dr. Golomb is the recipient of thousands of patient case reports on statin drug side effects.

Whereas Wolozin, et al., reported decreased prevalence of dementia associated with statin drug use,[7] Golomb countered in a letter to the editor of *Archives of Neurology*[8] that the Wolozin data could be taken to support a contrary conclusion—that high cholesterol protects against dementia. Golomb cited her many reports from statin users reporting cognitive loss frequently requiring medical work-ups for Alzheimer's disease and implying that the lowered cholesterol levels in such patients appeared to be a contributing factor. Her work is supported by Pfreiger's recent observation that Alzheimer's disease is characterized by a progressive and irreversible loss of neurons and synapses associated with cholesterol deficit.[9] Additionally, Henry Lorin, in his book, *Alzheimer's Solved,* has stressed the critical role of low cholesterol in the development of

Alzheimer's disease.[10] In light of this one can only shake one's head in wonder at the many studies planned or actually under way purporting to prove statins' benefit for this tragic condition.

That low or lowered cholesterol also contributes to aggressive behavior, violence, depression, and mood disturbance has led Kaplan at Yale University's School of Medicine and others to propose a cholesterol/serotonin hypothesis to explain the relationship.[11,12,13,14,15] Buydens-Branchey reported a strong relationship of low plasma levels of cholesterol and relapse in cocaine addicts.[16] Although the authors did not report specifically on the effect of cholesterol lowering medication on their patients, the inference is inescapable that such medication, especially with the statin class of drugs, might seriously aggravate the addiction problem.

As if the preceding were not sufficiently worrying concerning the hazards of low or lowered serum cholesterol, we have the report of Horwich *et al.*[17] that low cholesterol is a strong, independent predictor of impaired survival in older heart failure patients. From the work of Peter Langsjoen, we suspect a major contribution of coenzyme Q10 deficiency in these cases if such patients were on statins, but the authors caution that they did not have data on the patients' medical regimens. They imply, however, that low serum cholesterol is an independent marker of increased mortality in their patient group, suggesting mechanisms other than statin-induced ubiquinone deficiency.

Like many other, if not all, chemical constituents of our bodies, there may well be an ideal level of cholesterol in each of us. Low or lowered cholesterol, below our presumed ideal, "normal" range, and DNA mandated to be different in each of us, seems to be associated with a wide-ranging spectrum of problems from memory impairment, depression, suicide and dementia, to drug addiction relapse, and even with heart failure in the elderly. These observations are thoroughly documented and deserve thoughtful consideration by physicians prescribing statin drugs.

We will present more on the misguided war on cholesterol in the groundbreaking research of Dr. Kilmer McCully,[18] who further defines the innocence of natural cholesterol in favor of the culpability of homocysteine in the causation of cardiovascular disease as he points his finger at the true problem of atherosclerosis and scourge of strokes and heart attacks—inflammation!

CHAPTER 8
Inflammation and Atherosclerosis

No one has done more or worked harder in the past 40 years to determine the cause of arteriosclerosis than Dr. Kilmer McCully.[1] His persistent, pioneering research has revealed a wealth of knowledge about the process of this disease, the most common cause of premature death. Ignoring the huge tide of contrary medical opinion during that period, he insisted that there was more to the etiology of arteriosclerosis than high serum cholesterol, and he was correct as this chapter will show. Had the medical research field been receptive to his findings or even willing to consider causes other than cholesterol, the present flood of prescriptions for cholesterol-lowering statin drugs with their devastating side effects might never have occurred.

He had discovered that cholesterol comes in several different varieties. Some, known as oxycholesterol, contain extra oxygen atoms. Whereas pure cholesterol, free of all traces of oxycholesterol, is innocuous when injected into the arteries of experimental animals, oxycholesterol, obtained simply by exposing cholesterol to oxygen, becomes toxic and highly effective in producing arteriosclerosis in animals. Inflammation caused by this toxic agent could easily trigger a reaction resulting in elevated C-reactive protein (CRP). Natural cholesterol is innocuous. Oxycholesterol causes intense inflammation but this is not the end of the story. Now McCully had the reason why animals fed cholesterol in their feed got atherosclerosis but what about the results of autopsies done on Korean and Vietnam casualties? Most doctors were astonished to learn that the arteries of these 18 to 22 year old young men were laced with lipid streaks, foam cells and atheromatous plaques. Our story is now just beginning.

The United States of America was now about to embark on a three decade long application of the cholesterol/fat approach for the control of heart disease. Powered by ample federal funding, the bandwagon began to roll, carrying politicians, university administrators and directors of health departments and health agencies in its wake. These were the days of the Heart Disease, Cancer and Stroke legislation, which suddenly put universities into the healthcare delivery loop where a major effort was the promotion of cholesterol-control programs at community levels.

As physicians we began to write more and more prescriptions for cholesterol-lowering drugs. We lectured at service clubs and even to school groups on the benefit of cholesterol control and a fat-restricted diet. Any doctor not marching in this parade was considered academically deficient. Thoroughly endorsed by the medical and pharmaceutical establishments, cholesterol control drugs seemed to be the answer. These early drugs had side effects that were at times serious and even disabling, but the statin drugs were yet to be discovered and we encountered no amnesia, forgetfulness, confusion or disorientation.

Fortunately, not everyone accepted the cholesterol theory. Kilmer McCully, MD, working at Harvard during the late 1960s, had been involved in research that suggested a role for factors other than cholesterol and LDL in the etiology of arteriosclerosis. This was an almost inconceivable thought in those days. His interest was aroused when, as a member of the Harvard human genetics group, he was present when pediatricians presented the story of the death of an eight-year old boy, suffering from a disease called homocystinuria. The child had died of a stroke at that tender age.

This rare condition had been discovered only six years earlier by medical investigators in Belfast. In the ensuing years, several more cases were identified. In this condition, a genetic error occurs in a liver enzyme known as cystathionine synthase. When this happens, the amino acid, homocysteine, derived from the normal breakdown of protein in the diet, cannot be metabolized by the liver as usual and builds up to toxic levels. The arteries in these cases are abnormal, with hardening and loss of elasticity that greatly increase the tendency for heart attacks and strokes. Not only did McCully focus on this observation, but he also knew of the work of George Spaeth, an ophthalmologist friend, who informed him of the dramatically beneficial effect of vitamin B6 supplementation on some of the homocystinuria patients he had treated. Spaeth's homocystinuria patients often suffered from a dislocated lens. He reported his observation to McCully that the excretion of homocysteine in the urine of such patients frequently could be increased dramatically by vitamin B6.

Two seeds were firmly planted in Kilmer McCully's receptive mind: the amino acid homocysteine, if elevated, causes a condition remarkably like arteriosclerosis; and a simple vitamin, B6, could lower homocysteine levels. He was elated with this hint that a nutritional factor other than cholesterol might be involved, but his thinking was nothing more than a tiny candle lighting the darkness of lack of knowledge of this disease. He was alone with his concept and his original ideas fell on ears deafened by the roar of the cholesterol juggernaut.

McCully hurried to his laboratory and began to apply his skills as a pathologist to some of the original material from the homocystinuria case discussed at the genetics meeting. He found some paraffin blocks containing tissue from the young boy and a few of the original slides. Soon he was able to confirm that, indeed, the walls of the carotid arteries leading to the brain were severely thickened and damaged by arteriosclerosis, a form of hardening of the arteries. He now knew this disastrous blood vessel disease had caused the stroke that had killed the young boy. He found scattered, widespread changes in virtually all the small arteries of the body. He found neither cholesterol deposits nor plaques, just the routine calcified sclerosis and narrowing that he had come to associate with arteriosclerosis of the elderly.

Soon he had identified ten more cases of homocystinuria in children, many of whom had died of blood clots to the brain, heart and kidneys. All showed the hardening of the arteries and loss of elasticity associated with fibrous plaques. An abnormal reactivity of the blood platelets was evident in these patients, which accounted for the tendency toward formation of blood clots. Somehow, the presence of elevated homocysteine in the blood had caused the blood platelets to cluster more readily.

Sometime later at another genetics conference, McCully learned of another homocystinuria-like case: a two-month-old baby that had died despite aggressive attempts at therapy. This time, the urine contained both homocysteine and another substance called cystathionine, also related to homocysteine. In the case of this unfortunate baby, its metabolic passageway was deficient in a different enzyme and the conversion would have required vitamin B12. When McCully examined the slides of the baby's arteries he found the same arteriosclerosis changes noted in all the previous cases.

By now one should call McCully a medical detective, for that is what he had become. He admits he had difficulty sleeping for several weeks after this discovery because he knew he was on to something of extreme importance.

Like many scientists before him McCully had doubted the cholesterol hypothesis because cholesterol makes up so much of the human body and is so intimately involved in metabolism and physiology and cholesterol is a major component of the human brain. How could such a substance be sufficiently toxic to cause arterial damage? It did not make any sense to him.

Meanwhile it was now 1970 and researchers directed their attention to LDL in its Jekyl and Hyde guise, trying to understand why this innocuous substance behaved so erratically. In one instance it would provoke strong macrophage response leading to foam cell production, and at another time or in another form, its monocyte macrophages caused no pathological response.

McCully thought it likely that the receptor for LDL on the membranes of the endothelial cells lining the arteries was the determining factor and that the "activated" LDL, the process that makes LDL extremely "tasty" to a wandering monocyte, somehow takes place in these same cells. One wonders if this just might be where the lipoprotein (a) of Pauling and Rath[2] fits into the picture. First reported in 1991, this cholesterol carrying substance, so vital to arterial repair, had been routinely mistaken for regular LDL before then. The jury is still out on this idea, but research evidence is accumulating.

McCully lacked enthusiasm for the cholesterol/fat hypothesis prevalent in most of his co-workers. Not only was he drawn by the common sense appeal of his research-proven protein toxicity/vitamin deficiency theory, but he also knew the cholesterol hypothesis was lacking in several major respects. The most glaring deficiency of the then current cholesterol/fat hypothesis, according to McCully, was the fact that "the majority of patients with coronary heart disease, stroke and other forms of arteriosclerotic disease have no evidence of elevated cholesterol or LDL levels." [3]

McCully reported in his 1990 study[4] of 194 consecutive autopsy studies of mostly male veterans of finding only 8 percent of cases with severe arteriosclerosis that had total cholesterol levels greater than 250 mg/dL. He found the average blood cholesterol in the group with the severest disease was 186 mg/dL. This observation, perhaps more than any other, convinced McCully that medical researchers had to look elsewhere. The cholesterol/fat hypothesis provided no answers for this prevalent observation nor did it offer any reasonable explanation for how so ubiquitous a substance as cholesterol, a major and vital component of the human body, could provoke the onset of arteriosclerosis.

Another glaring deficiency of the cholesterol/fat etiology for arteriosclerosis was the observation, mentioned previously, from autopsies done on Korea and Vietnam military causalities. When one thinks about it, how could the extensive lipid streaks and early arteriosclerosis present in so many of these young men, many still in their teens, be attributable to a cholesterol causation when cholesterol/LDL levels in the young, supremely conditioned group were "rock bottom low?"

McCully had few allies during this time. Practicing physicians had a mindset created by decades of cholesterol/fat "brainwashing." The pharmaceutical industry had concentrated for decades on the development of ever more effective cholesterol control drugs. To say the endeavor was lucrative is a masterpiece of understatement. Billions of dollars yearly are involved; the profits are almost shameful in their excess. So the bandwagon had turned into a "cash cow" for the pharmaceutical industry and there were no friends for Dr. McCully there. Even the food industry would turn up its nose at a man who threatened their highly profitable, low cholesterol, processed foods and unsaturated oils by suggesting that relatively unprofitable fresh produce and, of all things, vitamin supplementation are healthy substitutes.

Finally, after "baiting the administrative lion for years" by investigating "dark alleys" and despite his 28-year affiliation, McCully's staff appointment ended December 31, 1978. One can only applaud the conviction of this man who, despite this setback, persevered. Gradually, as if to help McCully emerge from his doldrums, the seeds of a homocysteine causation of arteriosclerosis began to germinate and emerge from the research establishment.

Bridget and David Wilcken[5] began to publish their series of papers devoted to the study of homocysteine's role in heart disease. These doctors found that methionine given to patients with established heart disease resulted in large increases in serum homocysteine.

Many other epidemiological studies followed over the next two decades comparing the homocysteine levels of patients with heart disease, stroke, peripheral vascular disease, kidney failure, and even deep vein thrombophlebitis, with the blood homocysteine levels of normal controls. The current result of these studies is a consensus among medical investigators such as Boushey[6] that elevation of blood homocysteine levels is a strong independent risk factor for the development of arteriosclerotic disease.

The list of studies vindicating McCully's departure from established research pathways now goes on and on. Clearly,

Kilmer McCully was on to something back at Harvard when he was denied continued affiliation with their "forward thinking" research institution because "he had failed to prove his theory."

After years of study, the role of cholesterol in atheroma formation must be viewed as a passive one. There is now little doubt that a major cause of arteriosclerosis is the methionine/homocysteine metabolic interplay but other factors are likely to be involved. Even McCully will admit that adding together the possible contributions of hereditary predisposition, and even the most pessimistic estimate of dietary deficiencies of folic acid and vitamins B6 and B12 in the general public will not explain more than 40% of cardiovascular disease. Other researchers postulate that trans fats, grossly abnormal omega-3/omega-6 ratio, magnesium deficiency, inherent thrombotic tendencies, and even subtle anti-oxidant deficiencies, as possible contributing factors. Kauffman wrote an excellent review of this subject in the year 2000.[7]

Despite the glowing reports in the press, strong evidence exists that cholesterol levels do not matter. Ravnskov summarizes that statin drug therapy is reported to be almost as effective for high risk women as for men, despite the fact that most studies have shown that cholesterol is not a risk factor for women.[8] Additionally, the elderly with high risk are protected just as much as younger individuals, although all studies have shown that high cholesterol is only a weak factor for men older than fifty. Another observation mitigating against a cholesterol explanation for statin effectiveness is the consistent finding that strokes are reduced after statin therapy, even though high cholesterol is only a weak risk factor for stroke. Further confounding a possible cholesterol effect mechanism for statins is the fact that they protect regardless of whether the patient's cholesterol is high or low.

For these reasons cholesterol can no longer be cited as the sole cause of any patient's progressive arteriosclerosis any more than can smoking, hypertension, obesity or diabetes. It must be considered just another risk factor deserving attention. All of our present well-intentioned attempts at controlling cholesterol do little for the underlying arteriosclerosis or tendency for strokes and heart attacks.

So McCully has made a strong case for inflammation not cholesterol to be the culprit in cardiovascular disease and introduced the possibility that nutritional factors other than cholesterol are involved. There is now a compelling reason for radical change in the nation's diet and less dependence on pharmaceutical "crutches." To fight arteriosclerosis one must fight its cause. We need nutrition and health programs directed at such causes of inflammation as McCully's homocysteine, omega-3 deficiency and other arterial damaging factors that his research has led us to—the true causes of arteriosclerosis. Only in this way will we decrease our dependence on the statin class of drugs with their mind-robbing potential. We insist that transient global amnesia, permanent neuromuscular debility and profound behavioral changes are not acceptable drug side effects. But we must not lose sight of the fact that despite their many shortcomings, statins remain powerful anti-inflammatory agents and inflammation, it appears, is now the culprit. One might ask why we are still using cholesterol-lowering doses of statins when recent research points at inflammation not cholesterol as the real problem?

CHAPTER 9
The Misguided War on Cholesterol

A major part of heart attack and stroke prevention efforts these past several decades has been the so-called cholesterol-modified, low-fat diet. During this time, morbidity and mortality from atherosclerosis has changed little, if at all. True, through high-tech surgical intervention we have accomplished a miracle of restoring blood to threatened or damaged organs, but the prevalence of progressive arterial blockage remains largely unchanged. Apparently we have done nothing to stop or even slow down this dreaded condition. The burgeoning statin drug industry now feeds on nearly fifty million users and still, they say, we are not reaching all the people who should be on it. Some would call this medical progress, but I must call it a medical failure.

This quote is from Gary Taubes' very perceptive *New York Times* article, "What *If It's All Been a Big Fat Lie?*"[2] "If the members of the American medical establishment were to have a collective find-yourself-standing-naked-in-Times-Square-type nightmare, this might be it. They spend 30 years ridiculing Robert Atkins, author of the phenomenally best selling, Dr. Atkins' New Diet Revolution,[1] accusing the author of quackery and fraud, only to discover that the unrepentant Atkins was right all along. Or maybe it's this: they find that their very own dietary recommendations – eat less fat and more carbohydrates – are the cause of the rampaging epidemic of obesity in America. Or, just possibly this: they find out both of the above are true."

In 1972, just as the American Medical Association and the American Heart Association started the low cholesterol/low fat juggernaut on its fateful advance through the American public, a then little-known doctor by the name of Robert Atkins started his own trajectory, named *Diet Revolution*. He managed to sell millions of copies of his book by promising that a diet completely contradictory to the medical establishment recommendations was the way to go.

He promised the public they would lose weight by eating steak, eggs and butter to their heart's desire because animal fat was harmless. It was the carbohydrates—the pasta, rice, bagels, white and whole wheat bread and sugar—that caused obesity and heart disease, he contended. Atkins popularized his high-fat diet to such an extent that the American Medical Association considered his book and philosophy a threat to public health. Because of AMA pressure, Atkins was forced to defend his diet in congressional hearings.

The thrust of Atkins' diet and of the many similar carbohydrate restrictive diets that followed, of course, was to partake of foodstuffs requiring minimal insulin secretion, thereby tending to stabilize the hunger mechanism.

Since Atkins' debut in 1972, additional best selling diet books including *Protein Power*,[3] *The Zone*,[4] *Sugar Busters*,[5] Kilmer McCully's *The Heart Revolution*,[6] and others have polarized the American public on the subject of weight by recommending minor variations on the low carbohydrate/ liberal fat theme. All of them run contrary to the low cholesterol/low fat theme of organized medicine. The AMA preached that obesity and heart disease are caused by the excessive consumption of fat; the best sellers preached that carbohydrate is the villain and that fat is harmless. Despite the popularity of such books, the impact of organized medicine and the combined effects of the pharmaceutical and food industries have been far greater on the American public, and on all kinds of institutional food.

The result is the present obesity epidemic, our worsening incidence of Type 2 diabetes, and the realization that despite lowering blood cholesterols, the incidence of arteriosclerosis and heart disease differs very little, if at all, from thirty years ago. Some are finally ready to say the low cholesterol/modified fat diet has been an unhappy failure on the part of organized medicine.

Adding to this very real confusion, stirring the pot of conflicting ideology, so to speak, is the rapidly evolving reality that the notorious cholesterol may not be Public Enemy No.1, after all. Kilmer McCully's proposition that arteriosclerosis is largely an inflammatory response due to alteration in the homocysteine/methionine metabolic pathways with cholesterol assuming a passive role, at best, is rapidly gaining support. Although the jury still is out on this proposition, it begins to seem very likely that the medical establishment, fifty years ago, may have put all its many prestigious eggs in the wrong basket. If you want to go after atherosclerosis, place your sights on inflammation from homocysteine toxicity and nutritional deficiencies, not cholesterol. It seems impossible to believe that we have been wrong for all this time, but it is true.

Walter Willett, Chairman of the Department of Nutrition at the Harvard School of Public Health in Boston, reports from his comprehensive diet and health study,[7] the largest yet, that his preliminary data clearly contradict the low cholesterol/low fat ideology. In an ABC interview on 21st November, 2002, Dr. Willett stated, "The public has been told for many years that fats are bad and carbohydrates are good." This radical departure from current nutritional philosophy literally turns the USDA's food pyramid on its head. One can imagine the reaction of tens of thousands of well meaning dietitians and nutritionists to such heresy. To make matters even worse he added, "In fact, we've known for 30 or 40 years that that's not really true." Why, one might ask, was this respected and hallowed institution unable to muscle this information into national policy? Not only has our present nutritional philosophy failed to prevent coronary artery disease and ischemic stroke incidence but it also seems to have contributed directly to our obesity epidemic.

Next door, at Harvard's pediatric obesity clinic, David Ludwig stresses the negative impact of carbohydrates on insulin, blood sugar, fat metabolism and appetite—basic endocrinology apparently not fully appreciated thirty years earlier. To eat more fat-free carbohydrates inevitably leads to hunger and indulgence, then weight gain.

"For a large percentage of the population, low-fat diets are counter-productive," Taubes reports from his interview with the director of obesity research at Harvard's Joslin

Diabetes Center. "They have the paradoxical effect of making people gain weight."

How is it possible that a country like the United States has arrived at such a point where doctors who can find the time to consider and ponder such matters are beginning to feel uncomfortable and more than a little ashamed?

As Sally Fallon and Mary G. Enig have reported in their perceptive article, "*The Mediterranean Diet - Pasta or Pastrami?*"[8] It was Ancel Keys, then visiting professor at Oxford University, England in 1951, who first took note of the apparent benefits of the Italian national diet. He claimed this diet was characterized by abundant plant foods, fresh fruits and grains. As Professor Gino Bergami, Professor of Physiology at the University of Naples, reported to him at the first conference of the United Nation's Food and Agriculture Organization in Rome, "coronary heart disease was no problem in Naples."

Dr. Keys was intrigued with this comment and, shortly thereafter, he and his wife departed from their 1952 unheated apartment and the food rations of England to live for a while in sunny Naples. There, as a team, they studied this classic Italian diet but incorrectly deduced that it was low in fat, especially saturated fat. Serum cholesterol measurements of the local citizens seemed to confirm the apparent benefits. They concluded there was an association between diet, serum cholesterol and coronary heart disease.[9]

As Fallon and Enig reported, at first, Dr. Keys found little support for his revolutionary theories. But he encountered a sympathetic listener in 1952 when he presented his views to a small audience in New York at Mt. Sinai Hospital. Fred Epstein, convinced by Keys' data, began spreading the message "with great effect" over Europe and America. Keys expanded his studies and later, in 1970, published his Seven Countries Study,[10] in which it was later found that he had used selective data.[11]

After this research was published, the "Keys diet" became government policy and the darling of both the American Medical Association and the American Heart

Association. This was the well-documented and perhaps poorly defined origin of America's modified fat/low cholesterol rationale for national diet, which dominated scientific thinking and research for the next thirty years. Since that time unfortunate changes have occurred in the so-called Mediterranean diet. The food now served commonly is far from the former Mediterranean pattern. As Fallon and Enig so colorfully describe, "It must be distressing (for Keys) to observe sophisticated Italians feasting on such travesties as pasta Alfredo, veal scaloppini and prosciutto, especially to one who had taken the stringent vows of the diet priesthood."Study after study now finds the so - called Keys' Mediterranean diet largely a myth—probably a temporary result of the aftermath of World War II deprivation and half a decade of social conflict but one that became the basis of the low cholesterol/low fat diet.

Once the U.S. National Institutes of Health had signed off on the concept, however, the American food industry—suspected by some to be behind the whole thing— quickly joined in with a never-ending parade of reduced-fat products to meet the new recommendations. The fat content, which to a great extent gives processed food much of its flavor, was eliminated from many cookies and chips, ice cream, milk, cheese and yogurt and replaced by carbohydrates. These carbohydrates were inevitably the refined variety, relying heavily on refined sugar or starch, which, though adding bulk and perhaps taste, resulted in the public eating almost pure sugar, metabolically speaking. Aided and abetted by the missionary zeal of well-intentioned dietitians, health organizations, consumer groups and even cookbook writers, one could almost see America's waistlines expanding.

The impact of low fat/high carbohydrate diets on serum triglycerides was and is potentially lethal. By the late 1960s, triglyceride levels were already rising, protective HDL levels were falling and Type 2 diabetes was doing what it had to do —progressively rise. Endocrinologists like Gerry Reaven at Stanford University could see it happening. They even had a name for it - Syndrome X - but their voices could barely be heard over the roar of the low-cholesterol/reduced-fat avalanche.

And in the midst of all this "low cholesterol hoopla," drugs designed for the purpose of lowering cholesterol were to become the darlings of the pharmaceutical industry. Potentially, millions, then billions, of dollars of profit were to be made from statin drugs.

These same drug company researchers soon devised more and more effective statin drugs. In time, the truly effective ones—Baycol, Lipitor, Lescol, Pravachol, Mevacor, and Zocor—were developed, some capable of as much as a 40 percent reduction of LDL cholesterol in just a matter of weeks. More recently, Vytorin (Zocor and Zetia in combination) and Crestor have been introduced with an even greater claim for potency. So it has been only quite recently that these serious, even lethal, statin side effects have begun to emerge in a public and medical community lulled into complacency by ultra-positive direct-to-patient advertising and inexcusable misinformation.

The FDA prudently but somewhat belatedly "rushed" Baycol off the market after two years because of dozens of rhabdomyolysis deaths. Rhabdomyolysis deaths are still occurring, albeit at a much-reduced rate. Even so, the numbers of rhabdomyolysis deaths from Lipitor, Zocor and Mevacor, Pravachol and Crestor now far exceed those from Baycol alone. All of this for the purpose of lowering the blood level of the substance, cholesterol, that was already known to be absolutely vital for the human body to function. Even our very thought processes demand adequate supplies of this ubiquitous substance. Fully 1/2 pound of it is found in a 180-lb adult human body, much of it as fatty acid esters. And all of this pharmaceutical legerdemain is being done to control this wonder substance—which only occasionally winds up in atheroma because of misdirected "oxidized" lipoprotein—and which has no demonstrable causative role in atherosclerosis.

And now we find that such health care dignitaries as John Abramson MD of Harvard, Jerome Hoffman of UCLA and David Brown MD of Albert Einstein and Beth Israel, in a letter to NIH dated 23rd September, 2004, charged complete lack of objectivity of the originators of the latest NCEP guidelines due to financial ties with the drug industry and criticized these guidelines for gross lack of scientific validation. George Mann MD of the Framingham Study has previously called this misguided preoccupation with cholesterol causality "a cholesterol scam" and the "greatest scientific deception of our times." [12]

Cholesterol is not the enemy, inflammation is; and statin drugs, despite their benefit as inhibitors of inflammation, were designed originally to interfere with the mevalonate pathway and therein lay the problem. In inhibiting the mevalonate pathway of cholesterol synthesis, statins inevitably must inhibit our glial cell cholesterol, CoQ10 and ubiquinone, all so vital to the function of our bodies and minds—a terrible price to pay for inhibition of a substance now accepted by many to have no significant role in cardiovascular disease.

CHAPTER 10
A Failed National Diet. What Diet Then?

If the low-fat, low-cholesterol, all too liberal refined carbohydrate diet of the past 40 years has failed, leaving statin drug use and vascular surgery of one type or another at an all time high, where do we turn? What do we do? Our past leaders seem to have failed us. Who then is qualified to take the lead?

Dr. Kilmer McCully's far-reaching conclusion—that natural cholesterol is innocuous to arteries and elevated homocysteine, not cholesterol, is one of the major causes of arteriosclerosis—naturally led him to re-examine every facet of the prevailing public food habits. In regard to the FDA's diet guidelines, he unequivocally states: "The Food Pyramid is wrong on two counts: First, it is based on the false premise that cholesterol and saturated fats are the underlying cause of coronary heart disease. Second, it erroneously implies that all carbohydrates—whether refined or from whole food—are preferable to fats."[1]

One has but to look on the bookshelves of the local library and nutrition stores to observe that McCully is hardly alone in his philosophy. There are now many readable and informative books dealing with the subject of how our past decades of diet and nutrition standards have failed us. They very capably present the novel carbohydrate restrictive diet that McCully knew had to replace the old, national diet of the past. The first of these renegade leaders to gain notoriety was Dr. Robert C. Atkins but he was hardly the first to observe the problems inherent in the excessive reliance on carbohydrates in one's diet.

In 1862, the famous Dr. William Harvey imposed the then radical carbohydrate restrictive diet on his obese patient and friend, William Banting, with outstanding success. Banting lost over 40 pounds and, delighted, he wrote and published at his own expense his now famous *Letter of Corpulence*. Banting maintained a normal weight on his low carbohydrate diet until his death at 81.[2]

Atkins, a young cardiologist in 1963, found that for him a low carbohydrate diet worked to assuage his hunger and control his tendency to gain weight. He went on to write his famous book, on the protein augmented, carbohydrate restrictive diet.[3]

Atkins has been followed by legions of other writers rebelling against the guidelines and even the dictates of organized medicine represented by the United States Department of Agriculture (USDA), the American Diabetes Association (AdbA), the U.S. Food and Drug Administration (FDA), the National Cholesterol Education Program (NCEP), the National Heart, Lung and Blood Institute (NHLBI), and the Canadian Food Inspection Agency (CFIA). The millions of book sales these various authors have racked up against such odds reflect the awareness of the general public that all is not well with our food industry and national nutrition policies.

Joel Kauffman reviewed 12 of these popular books, comparing their strengths and weaknesses.[4] Kauffman describes the two books of this group which do not contain menus or recipes, one by Braly and Hoggan,[5] and one by Ottoboni and Ottoboni[6] as both excellent and complementary. He describes the homocysteine and oxycholesterol portions of the McCully and McCully [7] book as excellent and complementary to the foregoing ones. He praises a book by Bernstein[8] as being in a class by itself and must reading for diagnosed diabetics. For people not sure of which diet-based affliction they have, Kauffman encourages a book by Smith.[9]

For overweight people who want minimal reading and a simple diet plan to follow, the Allan and Lutz[10] or Groves[11] books are recommended. The Eades and Eades[12] and Atkins[13] books are for those seeking more information and diet plans. Kauffman even considers the special dietary concerns of those from Eastern Europe when he guides readers to a book by Kwasniewski and Chylinski.[14] In light of present knowledge, any one of these diets, if reasonably followed, will result in a general level of nutrition far superior to any served up by the low-cholesterol, low-fat doctrine during our past 50 years of homage.

And the slowly turning tide back to the natural fats that were the foundation of the American diet before the "prudent diet" became the national one is discussed in a paper by Mary Enig and Sally Fallon.[15] In "*The Oiling of America*" the authors offer a provocative and illuminating explanation of why the natural fats of our past diet—the butter, whole milk, lard and tallow—have been almost completely replaced in our society by the unnatural, highly processed vegetable oils loaded with the trans fats that are now competing with cholesterol as public health enemy No. 1, but happily, on their way out.

Of particular interest is Enig and Fallon's account of the famous heart surgeon, Dr. Dudley White, and his stance on the diet controversy. The "prudent diet" proponents of the low fat/cholesterol juggernaut crushed his 1956 nationally televised plea for nutritional common sense into oblivion. Dr. White noted that heart disease in the form of myocardial infarction (MI) was extremely rare in 1900 when egg consumption was high and corn oil was unavailable. When pressed to support the prudent diet, he replied, "See here, I began my practice as a cardiologist in 1921 and never saw a myocardial infarction patient until 1928. Back in the MI-free days before 1920, the fats were butter and lard, and I think we would all benefit from the kind of diet that we had at a time when no one had ever heard of corn oil." Today most people have forgotten all about Dr. Dudley White and his prophetic words of advice but we are now in a dietary revolution, and the natural fats of our grandparents are rightfully back in vogue.

However, the Heart Revolution Diet outlined in Dr. McCully's book, *The Heart Revolution,*[16] reflecting, as it does, his vast clinical research and conclusions, prompted me to focus on his dietary recommendations for the purpose of this book.

Dr. McCully's persistent, even tenacious, adherence to his almost "Eureka" concept of homocysteine toxicity causation of arteriosclerosis has gained wide acceptance from researchers in the field. From his first lonely review of arteriosclerotic changes in children who died from genetically pre-ordained homocystinuria, he now seems to have proven his point: cholesterol is not the cause of arteriosclerosis, inflammation is and homocysteine elevation secondary to vitamin deficiency appears to be a major player. Needless to say, to depart so radically from prevailing concepts takes a man with determination but it does not stop there.

McCully's historic work also points to vitamin deficiencies as playing the primary contributory role in arteriosclerosis. Homocysteine, the new villain, becomes predictably elevated in the body only when one or more of the B complex vitamins—folic acid, B6 or B12—are deficient. The arteriosclerosis of homocysteine elevation, it would seem, is a deficiency disease, which, according to McCully (and now many others) makes it potentially treatable by dietary supplementation. Cholesterol is not completely off the hook but its role, when sufficiently elevated, has now become one of passive incorporation into atherosclerotic plaque. Most authorities now accept these findings but are quick to point out homocysteine elevation, by itself, cannot account for all arteriosclerosis and atherosclerosis observed.

As presented by Fallon and Enig in their paper on heart disease causation[17] and Kauffman in his review on supplements,[18] other factors such as trans fats, unnatural omega-3/omega-6 ratios, insufficient magnesium, anti-oxidant deficiency, platelet malfunction, and even low levels of coenzyme Q10 may be involved. Certainly the concept of vitamin or mineral deficiencies as a cause or a significant contributor to public ill health is not new, but this major departure from traditional thinking, thanks in part to Dr. McCully's untiring efforts, now has widespread research support.

Now, another deficiency state with major repercussions must be added to the already long list of serious diseases now proven to come from a nutritional deficiency origin. Our big killer arteriosclerosis and its offspring, atherosclerosis, results from subtle deficiencies of such substances as folic acid, B6 and B12, the lack of which leads to toxic elevation of homocysteine levels.

McCully makes his case well, for these common substances—so vital to our ability to metabolize homocysteine—are not only exquisitely sensitive to the techniques of food preparation and processing but often become progressively less available to our bodies as we age. It can be stated unequivocally that despite the abundance of food in our burgeoning supermarkets, we are a nation in which many individuals are largely compromised by subtle deficiencies of folic acid, B6 and, particularly in vegetarians, B12. The result is rampant arterial disease with its heart attacks and strokes, our most common cause of death and disability. It seems ironic that a country so favored with such a rich array of resources can suffer diseases caused by something so prosaic as completely preventable vitamin deficiencies. Any doctor worth his salt in public health administration and delivery of health care cringes at the thought.

The FDA's inaction on the vitamin supplementation issues was another factor in my recommendation of McCully's *Heart Revolution Diet*. In his discussion of the carbohydrate restrictive diet, McCully devotes special attention to foods that have abundant amounts of folic acid and the B6 and B12 vitamins so important for holding homocysteine in check. He also advises the necessary cooking techniques that minimize the loss of these substances during food preparation. He generally goes along with the mid-section of the Food Pyramid but recommends a few modifications. Although milk, cheese and yogurt are good sources of calcium and protein and the recommendation to eat two or three servings per day is valid, he takes issue with the recommendation to eat only low fat or fat free products. He is concerned about the associated risk of deficiency of fat-soluble vitamins, since these nutrients are found only in the fat portion of the foods we eat.

Another area McCully would modify is the FDA recommendation to consume two or three servings of meat, poultry, fish, dry beans, eggs or nuts a day. Putting beans and nuts in this group is problematic, he says, because it suggests that plant and animal proteins are interchangeable: "The truth is that plant protein, lacking in some of the essential amino acids, is quite different from animal protein, which contains plentiful essential amino acids. Therefore, depending only on plants for protein is not a good idea because the protein is inferior." He suggests a daily intake of two or three servings of protein from fish, meats, poultry, eggs or cheese.

He agrees with eating more vegetables and fruits, which are an excellent source of vitamins, minerals, fiber and complex carbohydrates. He deplores the tendency of so many Americans to turn to highly refined, vitamin and mineral depleted, readily available, processed foods, which, for the most part, tend to be high in refined carbohydrates. As stated earlier, that excessive reliance on such carbohydrates in our diet has lead to the present carbohydrate catastrophe; the obesity epidemic.

McCully's diet is simple: Protein in the form of meat, fish, poultry, eggs, milk cheese and beans should comprise about 25 percent of our daily caloric intake. Another 25 to 30 percent of should come from the consumption of fats, which includes the fat of ingested meats plus olive oil, butter and cream. The remaining 45 to 50 percent of our daily caloric intake should be derived from the consumption of complex carbohydrates in the form of fruit, vegetables and whole grains. Balance is key in this diet.

You won't find white bread or French-fries in McCully's diet but you will find some remarkable similarities to the food nutritionists who postulate what our diet must have been like 10,000 years ago (although wheat would have been absent). Not only has McCully focused his diet on the prevention of arteriosclerosis but he also presents a diet to which we are already well suited, genetically speaking. We are still hunter-gatherers like our forebears, he says, but we must now confine our searches to the aisles of supermarkets in our quest for just the right foods.

Not only does McCully's diet help keep homocysteine levels comfortably in the normal range, lessening the possibility of damage to the lining of our arteries, it also seems to be just as effective for some as the low cholesterol/low fat diet for normalizing serum cholesterol, a subject of immense concern to today's patients, despite the lack of any significant association with cardiovascular disease. If one's arteries are not primed with lipid streaks and foam cells, LDL remains in its largely unoxidized form, and cholesterol deposition into incipient atheroma becomes unlikely.

The overwhelming majority of people today have been taught to regard cholesterol as the villain in coronary heart disease. Understandably, they have been led to consider the American Heart Association's low cholesterol/ low fat diet as the correct choice for keeping cholesterol levels in check. Because of this, they have become fair game for the promoters of broader and broader utilization of the statin class of drugs to reduce cholesterol levels. The reality that almost all major intervention studies have failed to find a significant correlation of serum cholesterol levels with cardiovascular diseases has fallen on ears deafened by drug promotional literature. Most individuals with the risk factors of hypertension, obesity, smoking and positive family history for atherosclerosis now consider themselves to be suitable candidates for statin drug intervention despite their frequently modest cholesterol and LDL levels. This makes the job of those promoting wider use of statin drugs even easier.

Now we have learned that cholesterol is not the villain in atherosclerosis, other factors are, primary of which is inflammation, secondary to homocysteine elevation among other causes. Our extraordinary efforts over the past fifty years to adhere to a low fat/low cholesterol diet appear to have been misdirected. This recent evidence suggests, even demands, a radical departure from our dependency on a misguided "national" diet that not only has failed to nourish and protect our health but also has actively undermined it. We need a new diet that is far more restrictive with respect to the consumption of carbohydrates and processed foodstuffs that have been stripped of vitally important vitamins and minerals. Authorities are surely beginning to realize that, had we taken this path fifty years ago, our current dependence on statin drugs for control of heart disease and stroke would be substantially reduced, if not eliminated.

It is for this reason that I felt compelled to include social emphasis on diet in my presentation of the diverse side effects of the statin class of drugs. McCully has given us reason to believe that, while cholesterol is an absolutely vital substance, it is innocuous in its natural, unoxidized form. Its passive involvement as a component in sclerotic plaques occurs only because of pre-existing factors completely unrelated to cholesterol. If we are to rationally approach the problems of prevention of atherosclerosis and its secondary complications of heart disease and stroke and excessive dependence on statin drugs, we need to recognize the full array of nutritional factors and inflammatory factors that are contributing. To accomplish this, anti-inflammatory supplements and proper diet must go hand in hand. Together, they can become a very effective "double whammy" in the prevention and treatment of atherosclerosis and its complications.

Applying these concepts one can look toward a future with a greatly reduced need for statin drug use. Our bodies are far too precious to risk compromise. Do we really have a choice?

CHAPTER 11
Enter Glyconutrients

Dietary supplements reviewed in this chapter have not been evaluated by the U.S. FDA for the possible benefits described.

The great variation of biologic properties that sugars offer to proteins as the peptide strands are being assembled is the strength of diversity, with virtually unlimited combinations of attachments thereby possible. Molecular biologists have calculated that four different amino acids alone can produce twenty four different structural combinations of the resulting peptide strand but with the addition of just four biologically active sugars with their multiple points of attachments there can result in one hundred and twenty four thousand possible structural combinations of the resulting glycoprotein strand. This incredible specificity of design is a major strength of sugars with each variation of structure allowing a functional change.

Another major area of sugar function is in cellular identification and cell signaling where sugar molecules on the cell's surface have the critical role of determining self from non-self, damaged versus healthy cells or inflamed tissue, which needs to be addressed. Our immune system is strongly dependent upon this role of sugars and so is the process of healing and regeneration.

Our neutrophils, macrophages and natural killer cells are the foot soldiers, our first line of defense against injury and infection. They use glycoprotein matching to identify problem cells. They attack only those cells not having proper ID. The chains of sugars extended from the surface of cell membranes is how the molecular identification is written for the white cells to read as "self" or "non-self." Our B-lymphocytes produce our antibodies and our T-lymphocytes engulf and destroy invaders much like our foot soldiers just mentioned but in a much more organized manner, seeking to destroy anything alien, again on the basis of improper glycoprotein ID. Even our cytokines such as Interleukin, tumor necrosis factor and interferons are dependent upon glycoproteins for activation. All of this has been thoroughly documented by research in which the necessity for one or more of the key saccharides has been shown to be absolutely essential.

Ordinarily, a normal healthy body produces its own supply of these biologically active sugars. Glucose and galactose are readily available in most diets and our bodies can convert them into the other sugars, but this conversion process is complex, energy dependent and prone to error. Many of us have lost key elements of the conversion process through disease or heredity or mutations resulting in a need for supplementation if our glyconutrient needs are to be met.

In these cases glyconutrient lack becomes comparable to the well-known deficiency diseases such as Beri-beri (vitamin B1 deficiency), scurvy (vitamin C deficiency), pellagra (vitamin B3 deficiency), anemia secondary to lack of iron and the huge goiters secondary to iodine lack. With glyconutrient lack, such persons become vulnerable to disease such as cancer and recover slowly from infections.

Of the many hundreds of research studies that have been done and are ongoing on the effects of glyconutrients on various disease states, including cancers of all types and AIDS and even respiratory tract infections and arthritis, all have been shown to benefit. I have referenced only a few to document the research interest that has arisen because of glyconutrients. A number of studies have shown tumor regression with glyconutrient supplementation.[1]

Glyconutrients decrease radiation sickness in animals and help them recover more rapidly.[2,3,4] Recent animal studies revealed that the mechanism whereby glyconutrients improve survival in their experimental mice with induced melanomas was likely to be by increasing T-cell and macrophage activity against their melanomas.[5,6] Two studies at Johns Hopkins have documented the ability of glyconutrients to prevent colds in children.[7,8] Certain rheumatoid arthritis patients have been shown to have a specific immunoglobulin dysfunction secondary to galactose deficiency. Treating these patients with galactose allows for the formation of normal immunoglobulin and relief of symptoms.[9] Recent research evidence shows that some children are born with a congenital inability to attach biologically active sugars to proteins. Such disorders are known as congenital defects in glycosylation. They are characterized by multi-system abnormalities. Central nervous system defects predominate. These conditions are uniformly fatal without glyconutrient supplementation. Their value in cystic fibrosis was reported by Vander-Wal, and Pippenger, in 2004.[10] Their survey went out to 271 families giving the supplements to their CF child with data showing improved quality of life is based on 98 complete responses. Dr. Pippenger is an award winning clinical researcher that pioneered drug blood level monitoring. Modest but definite responses in a complex area of use. Despite years of study on mechanisms of action of glyconutrients, the great complexity of our immuno-defense system is such that we are just beginning to scratch the surface of true understanding.[11]

Mechanism of action of glyconutrients

With considerable trepidation I now venture into the tiny microfactories within each of our cells where our biologically active sugars are attached to proteins. This is where glyconutrient supplements begin their metabolic journey. It is in the endoplasmic reticulum where the formation of glycoproteins begins. Of the two possible linkages of proteins to carbohydrates only the N linkage is important to us because only the N linkage demands the presence of the lipid known as dolichol phosphate (that statin suppressed substance I spoke of earlier).

This process begins with the entry of protein into the endoplasmic reticulum (ER) and continues throughout its passage into the Golgi cavity. Functionally this process closely resembles an auto body being placed on a modern assembly line to begin its conversion into a complete automobile. The core carbohydrate unit presented to the protein as it enters the lumen of the ER consists of three units of glucose attached to nine mannose units already connected to two N-Acetyl glucosamines attached to our dolichol phosphate "binder." Think of this as the installation of the engine complete with transmission. A wide variety of other sugars are attached to the carbohydrate core as it passes through the ER to the Golgi apparatus under the supervision of enzymatic attendants. Think robotic welders. When finally it arrives in the Golgi cavity, the resulting glycoproteins differ primarily in mannose content (horsepower?)

Now just say that dolichol phosphate is of poor quality or insufficient in bioavailability because of taking a statin drug. Our automobile will be dysfunctional because of trouble with the engine and transmission "binder." You now have problems.

Clearly, this description of the glycoprotein process, taken from Indiana University's internet biochemistry reference, suggests a primary role for mannose in this process but mannose never works alone. All members of the biologically active family of sugars must be available and sufficient in amount for the task at hand. Specific cases of galactose deficiency in certain types of rheumatoid arthritis already has been mentioned.

Another major area of glycoprotein function has to do with the glycoprotein molecules clustered on the surface of every cell in our bodies. The structure of these surface molecules is characteristic of that cell type and that cell type only, giving each cell a virtual identification tag. Not only is this the basis of our immuno-defense reaction, it is vitally necessary even in such a basic function as blood grouping. The key to blood transfusion is the ABO compatibility match between donor and receiver. The only difference between type O and types A and B is that the surface glycoproteins of type A and B contain one extra sugar molecule. Furthermore, the only difference between types A and B is in the sugar at one of the ends of the molecular complex. Type A has an extra acetyl group, lacking on type B. All are determined by glycoproteins.

Finally our glycoproteins are gatekeepers to the cells, regulating the transfer of ions of sodium, potassium, chloride and calcium through the cell membrane. Only recently has cystic fibrosis been identified as dependent upon a glycoprotein regulator responsible for the viscosity of the mucus within the tiny respiratory airways and pancreatic tubules.

Mention already has been made of the inevitability of dolichol inhibition by the use of statin drugs. This process, like CoQ10 synthesis, is not something that may happen when statins "gird" our mevalonate pathway, it is compelled to happen. Inhibition of CoQ10 synthesis by as much as 50 % has been thoroughly documented in research studies but measurement of blood or tissue dolichol remains currently impossible with today's technology and effect must be inferred by clinical observations.

There is no disputing the ability of statin drugs to inhibit dolichol synthesis and there is no disputing the important role of dolichol in the ability of our bodies to utilize glyconutrients. Therefore, impact on the mechanisms of glyconutrient action already described are inevitable. Of the three metabolic actions described for glyconutrients, that of dolichol supervised attachments of sugars to the growing peptide chain is of major concern for this is the stuff of neuropeptide formation. The types of protein and their sequence and folding characteristics are what determine the function of that particular peptide link. One combination gives love, another hate with hundreds of subtle values in between. Once formation of a peptide message strand is complete, the Golgi apparatus packages the product in a vesicle for safe keeping while traveling down the axon of a nerve to a synapse where they are stored until released. The ultimate effect of this magic cluster of chemicals owes much to specific sugars and their points of attachment. The makeup of the proteins is of vast importance, but it is the sugars which give it the rich spectrum of associated feelings, the subtle tones of guilt and fear that can accompany either love or hate. We human creatures soon come to understand our emotional complexity, our subtle interplay of grays on more gray. Rarely are things black or white. This is the music of our glyconutrient instruments, playing to their dolichol director. The contribution of just this neuropeptide role boggles the mind in its complexity and challenge to measure.

The effects on cell messaging and immuno-responsiveness are just as complex if not more so. At this point in our understanding it is impossible to predict the full spectrum of body systems potentially influenced by dolichols and glyconutrients. Even cognition and neuromyopathy problems may well be influenced. Only if apparently permanent side effects resolve with glyconutrient supplementation can we infer a cause and effect. We are in for surprises if we enter in to the definitive research to come with closed minds and fixed ideas.

We are now adding to our considerable base of anecdotal knowledge about glyconutrient effectiveness and, through the use of small pilot studies are beginning to investigate the effect of glyconutrient supplementation on statin users disabled by peripheral neuropathy, with the intention of following up with additional studies with statin associated chronic myopathy and ALS groups. Studies of this kind will lead the way to large double-blind, placebo controlled studies in the future to lay the firm groundwork required for more wide-scale therapeutic use. A positive factor concerning use of glyconutrients is that this is not treatment, but enhanced nutrition and there are seldom any adverse reactions.

CHAPTER 12
Anti-Inflammatory Alternatives to Statins

Dietary supplements reviewed in this chapter have not been evaluated by the U.S. FDA for the possible benefits described. This information is not intended to diagnose, treat, cure or prevent disease.

When confronted by the reality that one's statin is causing or might cause intolerable, even dangerous, side effects the question of alternatives inevitably arises. The usual course of action is to try another statin but only rarely does this resolve the problem for, regardless of drug company promotional hoopla, all statins are HMG-CoA reductase inhibitors and as such work only in one way—to inhibit the reductase step on the mevalonate pathway of cholesterol biosynthesis.

True, some statins seem more prone to one type of side effect than another but a dispassionate review of data shows them to be remarkably similar. Remember the Baycol rhabdomyolysis crisis? Baycol took the rap but rhabdomyolysis did not disappear, far from it. Now the combined numbers of rhabdomyolysis deaths from the other statins since Baycol's withdrawal far exceeds those originally caused by Baycol.

So, if another statin seems futile, what then? "What about my cholesterol and what about my risk status?" are questions frequently raised by anxious patients to their doctors. After 35 years of anti-cholesterol brainwashing, few people can easily comprehend that statins, originally felt to work solely as an inhibitor of cholesterol biosynthesis, now appear to work independently of cholesterol.

As I thoroughly discuss in my book, *Statin Drugs Side Effects,* statins work their magic of lowering cardiovascular risk not by cholesterol reduction but by their inherent anti-inflammatory action. Statins work regardless of cholesterol response. Despite this evidence of a new inflammatory factor in cardiovascular disease risk, the nutritional and pharmaceutical world remains steadfastly focused on cholesterol, the villain. The reasons are far more economic than public health oriented.

After believing the cholesterol myth for 35 years, the truth for me was not easy to accept. Nevertheless, anxious people must be told that it is not their cholesterol that determines their risk status, it is their personal and family history. Regardless of your cholesterol level, if your ancestors and blood relatives experienced premature heart attacks and/or strokes, you are at high risk. If you have experienced symptoms of angina, transient ischemic attacks (TIAs) or have a history of definite or suspected myocardial infarction (MI, heart attack), you are high cardiovascular risk and should be thinking "inflammation suppression." If statins at their traditional dosing levels no longer can be used, what then?

The Average Person

The focus should be on inflammation. Dietary means of inflammation reduction include common dietary supplements having proven anti-oxidant and anti-inflammatory action such as parent omega-3 with proper balance of omega-6 (see below for definition of parent omega), tocotrienol, vitamins B6, 12 and folic acid, co-enzyme Q10 and buffered aspirin. All of these readily obtainable, over the counter substances are of thoroughly documented benefit.

As to source and dose of the supplements, omega 3 is found in fish, especially the oil rich fish such as herring, mackerel, salmon (fresh and canned) and sardines. It is also derived from the krill of the northern oceans, available as a dietary supplement called krill oil. For omega-6 (in addition to omega-3) eat plenty of animal based protein like eggs, poultry, meat, cheese, yogurt as well as fish. Certain vegetable oils such as sunflower, safflower and walnut contain an abundance of omega-6. Flaxseed has far more omega-3 than omega-6. Fish oils are now increasingly available for use directly in capsule form containing the fatty acids EPA and DHA.

Tocotrienols come from grains, nuts and vegetable oils. Food sources such as palm, rice and annatto have the richest content of tocotrienols. However, these tocotrienols are often mixed with tocopherols. The only true source of tocotrienols is annatto, that is free of tocopherols. A typical 100mg tocotrienol dose is best to reduce inflammation, platelet aggregation, and adhesion molecules, all of which are responsible for atherosclerosis.

The 81mg dose of buffered aspirin is nearly as effective as regular aspirin in platelet inhibition (the mechanism of action of aspirin in CV disease) and has much less likelihood for side effects in unusually sensitive individuals. Remember the buffer contains magnesium, having its own benefit in heart disease.

For the vitamins, 80-100mg of B6, 200-250mcg of B12 and 400-800mcg of folic acid could be considered in the desirable range as a starting point for homocysteine control.

Dosage of CoQ10 depends on the condition and source (see ubiquinol). If you are using it with your statin merely to prevent the onset of muscles aches and pains or nerve damage, a dose of 100 to 200mg daily is reasonable. On the other hand, if you already have these problems and have stopped your statin drug and are trying to get back to normal, a daily dose of 500-1000mg might be advisable, especially since CoQ10 is a safe, natural substance. It is true also that in selected clinical trials of certain neurological diseases; doses up to 2,400mg daily are being studied. As to the best form, try to find gelcaps and look for economy.

a.) Omegas 3 and 6

Much has been learned recently about the omegas, 3 and 6 and their usefulness as anti-inflammatory agents. Until very recently the emphasis was solely on omega-3, portrayed as the omega of primary importance. This concept has recently been challenged by the results of recent research and much of the following is based on revolutionary work on PEOs (Parent Essential Oils). The physiologic and biologic importance of unadulterated parent omega-6 has turned out to be missed by most researchers in the field.

The inflammation suppression potential of the essential fatty acids (EFAs) has been found to be of such importance in arterial inflammation as to cause Lee and his group at the Thrombosis and Vascular Biology Unit of Birmingham's City Hospital in the U.K., to strongly recommend omega supplements in the long-term treatment plan of myocardial infarction patients. According to Lee, there is no longer any doubt as to the vital role of these polyunsaturated fatty acids in reducing cardiovascular disease risk. Recent studies have discovered that their strong anti-inflammatory effects are due to their ability to be converted into anti-inflammatory prostaglandins, also called eicosanoids.

There are two families of essential fatty acids: omega-3 fatty acids and omega-6 fatty acids. Both are termed "essential" because certain specific ones cannot be produced by the body and must therefore be obtained from the diet. Now we find that much of our ingested omega-6 has been inactive, rendered thus by food preservation, processing, storage and cooking so that EFAs are deficient both in amount and in ratio of one to the other, for omega balance is the key to proper metabolism. Now, nutritionists and physiologists are calling attention to this need for proper functional balance in the ratio of omega-6/-3 that we consume.

Now we are beginning to use the terms parent fatty acid, stressing that our intake must focus on the parent omega-6 (linoleic acid, LA) and parent omega-3 (alpha-linolenic acid ALA) that we eat each day, not their derivatives. So we shortchange ourselves when we buy derivatives, particularly when we focus on just omega-3.

Only recently have we learned how dramatically the ratios of omega-6/-3 have changed in meat and eggs since these animals no longer eat a variety of plants on the range but are penned and corn-fed. Adding to this has been the effect of modern food processing. Virtually every processed product on the supermarket shelves has been substantially altered, artificially, for increased shelf life, severely curtailing essential fatty acid amount and quality.

Now as to balance, we should be taking in nearly twice as much omega-6 as we do omega-3. This is a radical departure from what I have said in the past but it is based upon compelling research evidence. No longer do I recommend omega-3 supplementation alone. Modern food technology has changed all that.

It is true that the ratio of omega-3 to omega-6 in the typical Western diet has been falling for decades, closely paralleling the rise in heart disease during the same time period. However this has been accompanied by progressive deterioration in the quality of omega-6, especially due to the aforementioned factors of food storage, processing and cooking. A balance of omega-6 and omega-3 fatty acids is essential for proper health and we can achieve this only by supplementing our omegas together.

Research is still underway to define the precise mechanism by which these essential fatty acids exert their beneficial effect on reduction of cardiovascular disease risk. Our most important established truth is the now thoroughly documented role of EFAs in oxygen transfer. Oxygen from the blood diffuses readily throughout our lipophilic unsaturated fatty acids, transferring into our cellular mitochondrial membranes with ease. Both structure and function of the inner mitochondrial membrane and its four, protein/lipid respiratory chain complexes serve the need for oxygen transfer in ATP production. It reflects the perfection of evolutionary design.

A study published in *The Lancet* in March 2007 helps document the benefits of EFAs. This study involved over 18,000 patients with cholesterol levels deemed unhealthy. The patients were randomly assigned to receive either 1,800mg a day of EFAs with a statin drug or a statin drug alone. The trial went on for a total of five years. It was found at the end of the study those patients in the EFA group had superior cardiovascular function. Non-fatal coronary events were also significantly reduced in the EFA group. The authors concluded that EFA is a promising treatment for prevention of major coronary events, especially non-fatal coronary events.

The recommended dose of EFAs is quite variable, for there is no established upper limit to this vital food substance but balance is critical. My personal regimen includes at least 2,000mg to 2,500mg of omega-6/-3 supplementation daily as a routine, of which one third is parent omega-3 and the remainder is parent omega-6. Consider supplements as your insurance if you are at high risk.

b.) Ubiquinol – The CoQ10 of Choice

Peter Langsjoen MD, cardiologist, has been studying the CoQ10 supplement ubiquinol in patients with far advanced congestive heart failure. Many of these patients, because of the intestinal and liver swelling accompanying their congestive heart failure, often absorb coenzyme Q10 very poorly and will have relatively low plasma coenzyme Q10 levels on standard ubiquinone, regardless of dose. "We are seeing about a threefold improvement in plasma levels on equivalent dosages of ubiquinol in these critically ill heart failure patients. This improvement in plasma coenzyme Q10 levels has thus far been correlated with a significant improvement in their clinical status," Dr. Langsjoen adds.

Thus, ubiquinol appears to be lifesaving in patients ill with advanced heart failure. This form of CoQ10 can be considered mandatory in seriously ill patients or in those in whom regular CoQ10 has failed to help.

Following oral supplementation with the standard ubiquinone form of CoQ10, most of it is reduced to the usable form of CoQ10, ubiquinol, either during absorption or after the appearance of coenzyme Q10 in the blood. Ubiquinol accounts for more than 80% of the total ubiquinone and ubiquinol pool in human plasma, intestine, and liver. As you age, not only do you produce less CoQ10, but your body becomes less efficient at converting CoQ10 to the active form, ubiquinol. Over the past five years, scientists have discovered that higher doses of CoQ10 are needed to achieve optimal results.

This originally caused a dilemma with consumers, as they were faced with having to swallow many expensive CoQ10 capsules to derive the desired benefits. The ubiquinol form of CoQ10 is much preferred when higher doses are necessary to get the desirable blood levels. This product will cost you about triple, so use it only when the original product is inadequate for your needs.

The Higher Risk Person

For the even higher risk person, consideration must be given to even more powerful over-the-counter (OTC) anti-oxidants and anti-inflammatory supplements: vitamin D, tocotrienols and aged garlic extract (AGE). These substances may not be quite as familiar to you as the others but are thoroughly documented as to effectiveness. AGE has been around a long time. Tocotrienols will be new to you but I am personally convinced that when extra anti-inflammatory effect is necessary, they deserve special consideration. Everything that is done in public health and preventive medicine is based upon cost-effectiveness considerations, which means "getting the biggest bang for your buck."

Nowhere is this more true than for vitamin D. Only since 2004 has its powerful role in anti-inflammation been recognized. Just before then we learned of its vital role in cancer prevention, infection suppression and other immune system function. For 50 years before we knew only of its critical role in the regulation of calcium in our bodies and bone metabolism and I suspect there is still more yet to come from vitamin D.

c.) Tocotrienols, the New Vitamin E

Tocotrienols are naturally occurring members of the Vitamin E family. This is another one of those "medicine man" discoveries by Dr. Barrie Tan, who as a younger man exploring the jungles of South America, stumbled upon the annatto plant, primary source of this amazing fruit. This likable man is now busy introducing his discovery into broader use in the U.S. It is nice to know these chance encounters still can take place on our rapidly diminishing planet.

Dr. Tan says the annatto beans have been consumed by the Incas, Amazon rainforest dwellers and South Americans for several centuries where these tocopherol-free tocotrienols are intrinsic to their diets. All vitamin E molecules are antioxidants. Tocotrienols are much more potent than tocopherol, some 50 times more powerful. Many studies have proven that the annatto-sourced tocotrienols have superior potency.

For years tocotrienols have been overshadowed by the better known tocopherols, which long have made claim to the title, vitamin E. The truth is that the vitamin E in use these past decades has been tocopherol rich—and almost entirely alpha-tocopherol—and tocotrienol poor.

Recent research has demonstrated that tocotrienol rich vitamin E deserves another look for it has much greater effectiveness as an anti-oxidant with the added ability of modest cholesterol lowering, while at the same time raising HDL. It accomplishes this by its statin-like ability as an HMG-CoA reductase inhibitor while at the same time maintaining rather than blocking the mevalonate pathway. By far the most effective and potent tocotrienol compounds are the so-called delta and gamma forms.

Tocotrienols inhibit cholesterol synthesis by a unique ability to inhibit the farnesyl-PP to farnesyl step in cholesterol synthesis, bypassing the critical mevalonate pathway completely. Scientists have long sought a way to inhibit cholesterol at a point farther along the mevalonate pathway to avoid blockade. Tocotrienols accomplish this but their real strength may not be in cholesterol reduction, it is in their powerful anti-oxidant action.

Tocotrienols have shown significant tumor-inhibition activity in several studies involving breast, skin, prostate and liver cancer but it is in anti-oxidant, anti-inflammatory and neuroprotective effects that this product has demonstrated benefits far superior to tocopherols. They inhibit oxidation of unsaturated lipids in cell membranes as well as LDL cholesterol. They also inhibit platelet aggregation and activation while at the same time reducing monocyte adhesion and macrophage recruitment, the critical elements of the inflammatory response and the method by which statins exert their benefit in reduction of atherosclerosis and cardiovascular risk. In short they appear to have the benefit of statins with none of the risk of either excess cholesterol lowering or mevalonate blockade. Preliminary research is also looking positive for tocotrienols' ability to lower C-Reactive protein. This annatto derived product is obviously superior to all other forms of Vitamin E but contraindications concerning its thrombolytic action and dosage instructions must be followed closely.

Contraindications to Tocopherol-free Annatto Tocotrienol:
It may slightly potentiate the effects of anti-platelet medication such as Coumadin and Ticlid and it should not be taken with iron supplements.

Individuals on warfarin should be cautious in using doses of tocotrienols greater than 100 milligrams daily and, if they do so, they should have their INRs (International Normalized Ratios of prothrombin times) carefully monitored and their warfarin dose appropriately adjusted if indicated.

Likewise, individuals with vitamin K deficiencies, such as those with liver failure, should be cautious in using doses of tocotrienols greater than 100 milligrams daily. Tocotrienols should also be used with caution in those with lesions with a propensity to bleed (e.g., bleeding peptic ulcers), those with a history of hemorrhagic stroke and those with inherited bleeding disorders (e.g., hemophilia).

Tocotrienol supplementation (greater than 100 milligrams daily) should be stopped about one month before surgical procedures and may be resumed following recovery from the procedure. Preventing excessive platelet stickiness is how tocotrienols work in reducing cardiovascular risk, so do not let these warnings dissuade you. Platelet inhibition is vital to its role.

Those taking iron supplements should not take tocotrienols and iron at the same time as iron can oxidize tocotrienols to their pro-oxidant forms if taken together. Take iron supplements in the morning and tocotrienol with dinner. Proper dosage is important. Since tocotrienols can be converted to alpha-tocopherol in the body, taking too high a dosage of tocotrienols actually reduces their ability to lower cholesterol levels if this is the aim.

Typically 2 capsules deliver 100 mg of annatto tocotrienol (90% delta and 10% gamma) and was shown to have the maximum effect on reducing triglycerides and cholesterol and may prove more effective than higher dosages.

d.) Aged Garlic Extract (AGE)

The medicinal uses of garlic (Allium sativum) have a long history. Drawings and carvings of garlic were uncovered in Egyptian tombs, dating from 3700 BC. The major unique organosulfur compounds in AGE are water-soluble S-allylcysteine (SAC) and S-allylmercaptocysteine (SAMC) which have potent antioxidant activity. The content of SAC and SAMC in AGE is high because they are produced during the process of aging, thus providing AGE with higher antioxidant activity than fresh garlic and other commercial garlic supplements.

A substantial body of evidence shows that AGE and its components inhibit the oxidative damage that is implicated in a variety of diseases and aging. These effects strongly suggest that AGE may have an important role in lowering the risk of cardiovascular disease, cancer, Alzheimer's disease and other age-related degenerative conditions, protecting human health and mitigating the effects of aging.

Oxidative modification of DNA, proteins, lipids and small cellular molecules by reactive oxygen species (ROS) plays a role in a wide range of common diseases and age-related degenerative conditions. Oxidant damage by ROS is linked to photo-aging, radiation toxicity, cataract formation and macular degeneration; it is implicated in ischemia/reperfusion tissue injury and thought to play a role in decreased function of some immune cells. Antioxidants, including those in AGE, which protect against oxidative damage lower the risk of injury to vital molecules and to varying degrees may help prevent the onset and progression of disease.

To protect molecules against toxic free radicals and other ROS, cells have developed antioxidant defenses that include the enzymes superoxide dismutase, catalase and glutathione peroxidase, which destroy toxic peroxides. External sources of antioxidant nutrients that are essential for antioxidant protection include Coenzyme Q10, the antioxidant vitamins C and E, vitamin A / provitamin A and certain selenium compounds, a component of selenium-dependent glutathione peroxidase.

Phytochemicals from plant-rich diets, including garlic, provide important additional protection against oxidant damage. Studies in cell cultures of endothelia subjected to oxidant stress show that AGE protects endothelial cells from ROS injury by modifying cellular scavenging enzymes.

Nuclear factor-*kappa* B, the primary mechanism of action of statin drugs for cardiovascular disease reduction, is also inhibited by AGE. The antioxidative actions of AGE and its components are determined by their ability to scavenge ROS and inhibit the formation of lipid peroxides. AGE increases cellular glutathione in a variety of cells. AGE contains a wide range of antioxidants that can act in synergistic or additive fashion and protect cells against oxidative damage, thus helping to lower the risk of many chronic diseases as well as the tissue-damaging effects of ROS-producing radiation.

e.) Vitamin D

We are rapidly learning of the evolving roles of vitamin D in addition to bone metabolism and can even begin to postulate the reason for the development of such additional functions. The growth-arresting influence of 1,25-D on cancer cells makes sense in this light because excess UVB exposure is known to damage the DNA of skin cells, which can lead them to become cancerous. Some have also speculated that the antimicrobial response regulated by vitamin D is an adaptation that might have evolved to compensate for vitamin D's role in suppressing certain other immune system reactions—specifically, those that lead to excessive inflammation. As many of us know too well from experience, excessive UVB exposure causes sunburned skin, which at the tissue level results in fluid buildup and inflammation. Although a limited amount of inflammation is a beneficial mechanism for wound healing and helps the immune system fight off infection, too much inflammation causes its own havoc.

Perhaps not surprisingly then, an impressive body of work now shows that 1,25-D also acts as an anti-inflammatory agent that functions by influencing immune cell interactions. For example, different subtypes of immune cells communicate by secreting factors called cytokines to initiate a particular type of immune response. Vitamin D has been shown to repress exaggerated inflammatory responses by inhibiting that cytokine cross talk. Plentiful animal research has served to corroborate this.

This immune-suppressing function of vitamin D immediately suggested a range of new therapeutic possibilities for using vitamin D or its analogues in the control of autoimmune diseases thought to be caused by overactive cytokine responses, such as autoimmune diabetes, multiple sclerosis (MS) and inflammatory bowel disease. The RDI for adults in North America and Europe currently ranges between 200 IU and 600 IU, depending on age. Abundant evidence suggests that these values based on older concepts of function should be raised tenfold. Based on current information, doses of 3,000-5,000 IU daily seem entirely reasonable, especially when one is symptomatic for any of the conditions for which vitamin D may conceivably have a role.

Look for vitamin D supplements in the D3 form rather than the D2 form. Vitamin D3 (cholecalciferol) is the equivalent of what you would get from the action of sunlight on the skin and is up to three times more potent than vitamin D2 (ergocalciferol). Although sunlight on one's skin is an excellent source of Vitamin D, be aware that sunscreens, particularly the higher SPF numbers, almost completely block this process.

The Highest Risk Person

For the "highest risk" person, consideration must be given to the addition of statin drugs at low doses for their established anti-inflammatory benefit, but the dosage must be based on reduction of inflammation, not cholesterol.

f.) Low Dose Statins

This may be surprising to some but after thorough research of this subject I consider low dose statins to be a rational part of this section.

From the very beginning of statin use, dosing at cholesterol lowering doses has been the standard. Statin dosing should be at a dose that will address inflammation without the inevitable mevalonate blockade of conventional dosing, for with mevalonate blockade comes the side effects. Hilgendorph laid the groundwork for this concept in his use of inflammation as a marker of statin effect, finding surprising robust anti-inflammation with low dilutions of statins and only minimal increases in effect as concentrations were increased.

As I discuss in *Statin Drugs Side Effects*, much more study is necessary to validate the concept of low dose statin dosing. Much information already is available suggesting that dosages required for effective inflammation reduction are much less than that required for cholesterol reduction. My personal choice would be Pravachol 5mg, or 2.5mg/day if stronger statins such as Mevacor, Zocor, Crestor or Lipitor are used.

g.) Red Yeast Rice

I might also suggest investigating the use of red yeast rice at the low dose of one 500-600 mg capsule daily (remember that dosage of active ingredients in Red Yeast Rice may vary considerably between brands—generic lovastatin is more reliable in dose). Individual sensitivities to a drug or supplement can vary widely. I am certain my preferences are biased by my personal experience of Transient Global Amnesia associated with a 5mg daily dose of Lipitor for 6 weeks.

h.) Diet

As to diet, I personally try to follow a mostly paleolithic diet with its ideal omega-3/omega-6 ratio from plants, nuts, vegetables, fish, farm eggs and pasture-raised meats. All others should refer to my comments on the *Heart Protection Diet* based on Doctor Kilmer McCully's informative book, *The Heart Revolution,* and pattern your eating habits after it as much as possible. And do not forget to exercise.

CHAPTER 13
Failure of MedWatch

Only a small percentage of adverse side effects are reported to MedWatch. Estimates for reporting of adverse drug reactions (ADRs) range from 1% to 10% meaning that the actual number of adverse reactions could be at least ten times higher than those reported to MedWatch.

This is MedWatch, the U.S. government's protective umbrella, supposedly shielding us from adverse post-marketing drug events, but actually completely subservient to the drug companies in that money for MedWatch salaries comes from drug company pockets.

And to think about how little of this information is known to practicing physicians. Hardly a day goes by that I do not get a report or two from doctors saying, "I didn't know statins could do that," and this years after my own experience with Lipitor associated amnesia. "Statins don't do that" was a refrain I heard over and over again from both doctors and pharmacists as I sought answers to my two statin associated amnesias. During the first episode at 10 mg daily, I retrograded back ten years and, for six hours, knew neither my new wife nor my new home. In my second case at 5 mg daily, I was 13 years of age for 12 terrifying hours and laughed hysterically when they told me I was married with children and a family doctor. I was 13!

I attended a shipboard medical seminar where the fully credentialed cardiologist who was giving the credit course told me he had never seen a case of memory problems or amnesia in someone on a statin drug. He was amazed and completely unreceptive when I gave him a few statistics. And what about huge clinical studies wherein thousands of participants are placed on today's heroic doses of statins with nary a problem according to the investigators.

Pfizer's own statistics tell us to expect five cases of amnesia for every one thousand statin users. Who is doing the monitoring of these studies for side effects? What questions are being asked? If neither doctor nor patient knows that memory lapses are possible in statin users, how often will it be reported? I can only surmise that cognitive side effects from statin drug use are not being seen because they are not being looked for.

At the very heart of the patient/clinician relationship there should be trust that the doctor is fully informed about the drug he or she is using or preparing to use. This seems elementary yet the medical community appears almost completely uninformed about statin drug side effects. How then can these same physicians be trusted to explain potential problems to the patients?

The first time I was given Lipitor I experienced a six-hour episode of transient global amnesia. When I suggested, on the basis of my 23 years as a family doctor, that perhaps my new medicine was the cause of my amnesia, the neurologist replied, almost scoffingly, that "Statins do not do that." He and many other physicians and pharmacists were adamant that this does not occur.

A neurologist insisted I continue on my Lipitor. The next day during my MRI, I had occasion to talk of this with other doctors and pharmacists all of whom said, "Statins do not do that." They clearly seemed surprised that a physician apparently of sound mind and body would even consider such a thing. Being master of my own ship, I stopped my statin.

After an uneventful year I returned to Johnson Space Center for my repeat annual physical where I was told, yet again, after describing my episode that, "Statins did not do that and I must go back on my statin." With considerable reluctance but no confirmation from any doctor or pharmacist the previous year, I agreed to restart my statin at one-half the previous dose. After about two months I had my second, much worse attack of TGA, lasting for 12 hours during which time my entire adult life had been eradicated. NASA still insisted this was no more than a strange coincidence and were adamant that they had no reason to change their ongoing practice of prescribing statins for simple modest hypercholesterolemia. Even then after my second bout with TGA from Lipitor, I remained the only one convinced of the relationship.

You can imagine how disgusted I was later to learn about the 11 severe cognitive dysfunction cases in Pfizer's 2,503 volunteer patients. To me that incidence of 4.4/1,000 cases of severe memory impairment associated with the use of Lipitor was highly significant.

Management had decided to ignore it, helping greatly to explain the reaction of my colleagues at FAA headquarters and the Pentagon later when I told them of my experience. As a flight surgeon for several decades I knew the special importance of this in the case of pilots and I had heard that both of these organizations were allowing pilots to fly with statins. You can guess what my colleagues said – "Statins don't do that."

In my review six years ago of MedWatch data from 1997 to 2006, I reported finding 662 serious cognitive loss problems, just from this one statin alone and they all do it![1] At no time in the last decade has the FDA seen fit to report this to the practicing physicians out there, and the same situation holds for the entire range of statin drug side effects, whether rhabdomyolysis, peripheral neuropathy or neuromuscular degeneration.

The facts remain that vital information about the frequency of cognitive impairment, permanent peripheral neuropathy, chronic myopathy and chronic neuromuscular degeneration has been locked up in MedWatch for nearly a decade under the guise of "being studied."

Can you imagine the effect on marketing if word got out that for every one thousand people on a statin, five cases of abrupt cognitive impairment and amnesia will occur. Or, for myopathy with its aches and pains, whether CPK is normal or elevated, 25% will be permanent?

The overwhelming majority of physicians in the United States today are completely uninformed of the true legacy of statins. This is why I make my strong case that our physician caregivers cannot possibly give us informed consent when they haven't the slightest idea of the truth.

As documentation of exactly where we are today on the subject of the FDA reporting back to physicians, I have taken it upon myself to do an actual count of all relevant MedWatch data for the statin drug Lipitor from the period 1997 to May, 2012.

Adverse Drug Reports for Lipitor (atorvastatin) (From 1997 thru 15 May 2012)

I was last able to access MedWatch data in 2006. The process had not been easy for it meant I had to tackle the immense challenge of reviewing manually some 64,000 Lipitor Adverse Drug Reports (ADRs) using "find" on my computer. What prompted me to do this personal search of what most would agree is the FDA's business, is the almost total lack of awareness by doctors of statin associated cognitive dysfunction, emotional and behavioral disorders and cases of disabling neuro-muscular degeneration. Clearly doctors have not been informed. Yet I know of the many thousands of MedWatch reports that have been submitted. In some cases I have been instrumental in helping distraught victims make their MedWatch report.

Based upon my personal cognitive experience with this drug, amnesia was the first search term I entered. Not unexpectedly, out popped 1,302 case reports for amnesia in the MedWatch files. Adding the search term "memory impairment" added another 663 cases. This gave a total of 1965 reports of serious cognitive dysfunction associated with the use of Lipitor.

A word of caution concerning gross under-reporting deserves to be mentioned here. First of all, anyone experienced with the operation of such optional reporting systems as MedWatch fully realize that the results are but an approximation of the actual numbers. Estimates for reporting of adverse drug reactions (ADRs) range from 1% to 10% meaning that the actual number of adverse reactions could be ten to a hundred times those reported to

MedWatch. Additionally, only the more severe forms of cognitive dysfunction get reported—the transient global amnesia and severe memory loss cases. Rarely included, and therefore expected to be missed, are the more minor forms of cognitive loss such as confusion and disorientation and unusual forgetfulness.

Then we have the category of short term cognitive loss with durations measured in seconds and minutes that by their very nature will rarely be recognized even by the victim, say nothing of an observer, yet might be so critical to a pilot. The passage of time is too short for recognition yet special studies have revealed just how common they can be. Despite the fact that in February, 2012 the FDA for the first time announced cognitive dysfunction as a major side effect of statin drugs, they immensely under-played its seriousness. At no time did they even mention transient global amnesia; a strange form of completely incapacitating amnesia in which the victim abruptly, without the slightest warning, loses the ability to formulate new memory, accompanied by retrograde loss of memory for decades into their past. The past decade has seen a big increase in reports of this once rare condition. They instead mentioned some transient episodes of confusion and disorientation might occur that usually were mild and passed with no complications. Never a word was said about the possibility of a military or civilian commercial pilot suddenly encountering this form of amnesia with retrograde loss of their flight training. It is not only pilots that need to worry. This concern applies to anyone whose occupation requires extra vigilance including professional drivers, heavy equipment operators, surgeons, military personnel, etc.

Applying additional cognitive search terms gave me 222 reports of "dementia," 523 case reports of "disorientation" and 602 reports of "confusional state." I next searched among words that might reflect the curious effects of statin drugs on emotion and behavior now being reported. I found 347 reports using the search terms "aggressiveness," "paranoia" and "irritability" commonly reported in statin users.

Use of the search term "depression" yielded 1,142 reports of which 118 expressed "suicidal ideation."

Since it also was in February, 2012 that FDA first mentioned the persistent seriousness of rhabdomyolysis, that was the next search term I entered. Rhabdomyolysis is an especially serious form of muscle damage with a fatality rate of 10%. You may recall that it was rhabdomyolysis that brought down cerivastatin (Baycol) with some 60 deaths in the year 2004 causing Bayer to remove it from the market. Deaths in these cases are due to kidney failure caused by the blockage of renal tubules by fragments from damaged muscle cells that have been carried to the kidneys in the bloodstream. I counted 2,731 MedWatch reports of rhabdomyolysis. Removing Baycol from the market in 2004 did not stop the statin-associated loss of lives from rhabdomyolysis. Lipitor quickly filled this void and similar rhabdomyolysis death rates can be expected from the other strong statins. I calculate that each year Lipitor accounts for more than 20 deaths from rhabdomyolysis. Applying additional search terms bearing on the muscular system I found 1,325 reports of "myalgia" and 494 reports of "musculoskeletal stiffness." Applying the search term "renal failure" gave me 2,240 responses, comparing favorably with the 2,731 MedWatch reports of rhabdomyolysis cases, knowing that many, if not most, of these would be accompanied by varying degrees of renal involvement.

Being well aware of the great numbers of reports of peripheral neuropathy in my repository, the next term I chose was "neuropathy" which yielded 1,294 reports to MedWatch. It should be mentioned that almost all of these peripheral neuropathy reports have proven to be very resistant to traditional treatment and many now deserve to be called permanent. Using the term "Guillain-Barré syndrome"—a disorder affecting the peripheral nervous system—gave 98 reports, and prompted by hundreds of case reports I have received complaining of leg and arm pain, the search term "pain in extremity" gave 3,498 reports.

Next I put in the search term, "hepatitis." Before I tell you the number, I first must qualify it by warning you that there are many different kinds of hepatitis. There is hepatitis A, B, C, cholestatic, autoimmune, fulminating, acute, chronic and viral, including cytomegalovirus. All of these terms are used in this compilation of Lipitor damage reports. However, the overwhelming majority of these reports said simply, "hepatitis" with no qualifier. Since hepatitis has always been a warned concern from statin use you must make up your own mind in interpreting the 2,102 total cases that resulted. When I realized that "liver function abnormalities" also was being used in the MedWatch diagnoses list, I used it as a search term, reporting 842 liver function abnormalities in addition to the 2,102 hepatitis cases for a grand total of 2,944.

I should add here my thoughts on the way liver function test guidelines have been grossly manipulated during the statin era. Some twenty years ago, doctors were still advised to use the guidelines that I had been accustomed to since my medical school training. Now, starting close to 1990, the time when statin use began to get seriously underway, doctors were asked to replace their usual routine of using the mean plus 2 standard deviations (SDs) with the mean plus 10 SDs to determine when an elevation of liver enzyme due to statins was significant or not. This incredible distortion of reality was done in order that we not get too excited about 2 SDs when dealing with statins. The previous guidelines no longer applied. I am still trying to figure out how the clinical pathologists got away with that. It made no sense then and much less sense now. Inflammation is inflammation. When dealing with statins we have been asked to accept small amounts of inflammation as normal.

Since the unexpected association of amyotrophic lateral sclerosis (ALS) with statin use was reported by Ralph Edwards of the World Health Organization using their VigiBase® data, my next investigation of Lipitor MedWatch data was for search terms that might give a measure of ALS occurrence. "Unusual weakness" turned up 2,516 case reports, "balance disorders" gave 596 responses and "coordination abnormalities" gave 195 responses. Since I have this condition I can speak with authority on the subject of balance disorders. A kindly neighbor lady was so concerned on seeing me walk by her home she offered to drive me the rest of the way. Until that moment I was unaware of the effect of my walking on the public eye. Clearly this "Good Samaritan" sensed me as disabled. My transition to a walker frame took place the following day.

Relevant to diabetes, in a recent article in the *NEJM* http://www.nejm.org/doi/full/10.1056/NEJMp1203020 a meta-analysis of six statin trials is referenced that revealed a 13% increase in the relative risk of new-onset diabetes in those taking a statin. The FDA also added an increased risk of developing Type 2 diabetes to their February 2012 warnings—an amazing side effect for a medicine that is supposed to diminish the risk of cardiovascular disease. I used the search term "pancreatitis" to see how much of this diabetes might reflect organ damage. I found 604 reports of pancreatitis.

I see this as part of a whole body process of mitochondrial DNA damage aggravated by the use of statins. Even on our good days, mitochondrial mutations occur by the tens of thousands leading to progressive mitochondrial loss followed in time by cell loss and finally, with sufficient time, organ damage in the well known process of aging. All of this is the inevitable consequence of normal metabolic activity. It is theft of electrons from adjacent tissues, including DNA strands, that causes the damage. CoQ10 plays a major role not only in energy formation via electron transfer but also anti-oxidation, minimizing buildup of oxidizing byproducts of metabolism and slowing down DNA damage. Via inhibition of CoQ10, statins play a major role in what amounts to enhancement of the aging process.

Applying the search term cancer (of all kinds) gave me 1,642 official reports to MedWatch of which 422 were reported as breast cancer. I next tried the search term "cardiac failure" and turned up 720 reports. CoQ10 inhibition is felt to be the major contributor to this condition. My next search was "myocardial infarction"—out of curiosity—to see how many might there be in a group already on Lipitor. The figure was 2,520—another attention getter, especially when I got 610 additional reports using the search term "coronary artery occlusion." When you get a total of 3,030 cardiac events in a group already on statins you are justified in wondering just how much protection is being offered? Use of the search term "cerebrovascular accident" (a stroke) yielded 1,562 reports with another 159 inferred by the use of the search term "aphasia."

My last search focused on tendon complications. I found 436 from Lipitor over the time period of this report. This relatively obscure finding is based upon the role of cholesterol in tendon and ligament function. Most orthopedic surgeons are well aware of this relationship.

The FDA has a first rate monitoring system but a grossly deficient one for reporting findings back to the medical community. The average primary care physician in the U.S. today, knowing that perhaps only 10% of patient problems get reported to the FDA, would be startled to see these figures, especially the ones for cognitive dysfunction, neuropathy, rhabdomyolysis, depression, neuropathy and hepatitis. These are the people who write the prescriptions for statin use.

CHAPTER 14
Serious Statin Drug Side Effects

a.) The ALS / Statin Link

My statin drug side effects repository grew during the past ten years as a result of my own experience with statin associated amnesia and the associated media attention. Just a few years ago, the numbers of case reports of amyotrophic lateral sclerosis (ALS - known also as Lou Gehrig's disease) was a trickle; now it is a relative flood.

There is not the slightest doubt in my mind that the numbers of reports I am seeing now are far more than usually expected in a group the size of my reporting population. One naturally wonders about this curious relationship with statin drugs and what the possible mechanism of action might be?

Neuroscientist, V. Meske[1] reported in the European Journal of Neuroscience a very relevant study about the ability of statin drugs to cause neuronal degeneration. To refresh your memory statin drugs are designed to inhibit cholesterol synthesis by their effect on the mevalonate pathway. It seems that a consequence of the inhibitory effect of statin drugs on the mevalonate pathway is the induction of abnormal *tau* protein phosphorylation. *Tau* protein phosphorylation goes on to form neurofibrillatory tangles, long known to be the prime suspect in causing the slowly progressive neuronal degeneration of Alzheimer's disease. Sometimes this process is accompanied by Beta amyloid deposition but more commonly not. Research scientists are now finding that this mechanism appears to be true for ALS and many other forms of neurodegenerative diseases as well. They have even coined a new word for this, the taupathies.[2,3,4,5] Included therein are: Amyotrophic Lateral Sclerosis (ALS), Parkinson's Disease (PD), Frontal Lobe Dementia (FLD), Alzheimer's Disease (AD) and Multiple System Abnormalities.

Statin associated taupathies may well be additional gross evidence of collateral damage to existing cellular chemistry that researchers were unable to predict when they originally developed the statins. The possibility of mitochondrial mutations has also been cited as a possible mechanism of action for the induction of ALS or ALS-like conditions. And it might well be that more than one mechanism may be involved. All this from a class of drugs originally designed simply to inhibit the biosynthesis of cholesterol, a vital substance now apparently irrelevant to the atherosclerotic process.

Very few primary care physicians are familiar with the association of statin drug use with ALS and most are disinclined to use warnings from websites about statin drug side effects, saying they are anecdotal. These "anecdotes" are the patient's histories! Doctor Ellsworth Amidon, my Vermont College of Medicine professor of medicine, used to say, "Heed well the words of your patients, my young doctors, they are telling you the diagnosis."

Most physicians feel that the pharmaceutical industry is on guard for side effects such as this and if no black box warning is out, the drug is safe. This is terribly naïve. Nor is the FDA's MedWatch an effective monitor of drug safety. My personal experience with MedWatch is that it is an adequate repository only. As an example, primary care physicians were denied the existence of statin associated amnesias until Wagstaff *et al.* reported in *Pharmacotherapy* their 60 cases gleaned from a MedWatch review in 2003.[6]

Additionally my own review of MedWatch data (see previous chapter) reveals many hundreds more statin associated TGA cases that no one at the FDA has reported back to our physicians. I can only hope that readers of this book, especially those having relevant symptoms, will bring this subject to the attention of their doctors.

All reductase inhibitors—statins—have the potential for collateral damage to existing mevalonate cellular chemistry with inhibition of dolichol, CoQ10 and glial cell cholesterol synthesis. This potential for damage is all but inevitable with reductase inhibition at the mevalonate to mevalonic acid step, causing what amounts to a mevalonate blockade. Statin associated taupathies may well be additional gross evidence of collateral damage to normal phosphorylation chemistry that researchers were unable to predict when they originally created the statins. All this from a class of drugs originally designed simply to inhibit the biosynthesis of cholesterol, a vital substance now of questionable relevance to the process of atherosclerosis.

In some of these ALS or ALS-like cases, individuals have reported to me that symptoms have regressed after stopping of the statin drug, lending credence to possible statin drug causation. In other cases various supplements have been utilized in addition to stopping the statin drug, with varying degrees of improvement in the clinical picture.

Sharing of Statin/ALS Experiences

The People's Pharmacy® website carries an unexpected goldmine of ALS incidence data in a page titled *Statins and ALS-Like Syndrome.*

http://www.peoplespharmacy.com/2009/07/31/statins-and-als/

Joe Graedon started this page in 2007. In it he has invited anyone struck down by statins with symptoms suggestive of ALS to comment on their status for the benefit of others.

Although the Graedons were aware of muscle problems as well as nerve issues (peripheral neuropathy) associated with statin drugs, they had not heard of ALS cases linked to these medications. Then they received an email from a reader of their syndicated newspaper column: *"I read with interest today's letter from a Lipitor taker. I believe Lipitor triggered my ALS, but had a hard time convincing anyone until this World Health Organization report came out."* They decided to post an ALS/statin drug statement inviting readers to report relevant experiences. Their invitation read: *"If you have an experience you would like to report about statins in general or an ALS-like syndrome in particular, please write about it here. We will pass on your case report to the FDA."*

The result was astonishing! Over the next three months many hundreds of case reports came in from which seventy two presented with the constellation of symptoms usually associated with ALS but the official diagnosis had not yet been made. I termed these, ALS-like. Additionally well over a hundred reports came in from people experiencing peripheral neuropathy, the other symptom complex reported by the WHO to appear in excess numbers worldwide in those on statins.

b.) Permanent Peripheral Neuropathy

I have received hundreds of emails and letters from diabetic patients confused by their doctor's insistence on putting them on statins. Peripheral neuropathy was reported by the World Health Organization's VigiBase as being excessive in statin users worldwide (along with amyotrophic lateral sclerosis). Frankly, I am as confused as these diabetic patients and would consider the presence of diabetes to be a contraindication to the use of statins unless low, anti-inflammatory doses are used. In this manner they would get a reasonable reduction in inflammation with very little risk of mevalonate blockade, the cause of most of the side effects. Who gets the blame for the neuropathy that is almost certain to develop with higher doses?

Now let's take another look at peripheral neuropathy. Yes, drug companies have listed peripheral neuropathy in their long list of adverse warnings posted in every doctor's *Physician's Desk Reference*, but here they forgot to say one thing— they never said that peripheral neuropathy was going to be permanent and almost completely unresponsive to treatment. Rare it might be but I know of some 250 statin victims in walkers and wheelchairs because of the association of nerve damage with statin use.

Thus far we had recognized that statin associated peripheral neuropathy was permanent. Most people with this condition had already been through the ropes with test after test by specialist after specialist. None had the slightest appreciation for the reality of statin causation and in almost all cases it was a diagnosis of frustration; the last possible cause they would consider and most preferred etiology unknown. Once these patients went through the diagnostic hurdles, they then had to overcome the treatment hurdles before finally realizing that nothing helped them. Traditional medicine had nothing to offer. Their backs were to the wall. Previously fully functional people were now considering the use of wheelchairs and the painful process of seeking other employment.

It should be noted that excess numbers of peripheral neuropathy cases were noted and reported from the World Health Organization as well. Referring to Chapter 13 of WHO VigiBase reported that of a total of 5,534 individual case reports of peripheral neuropathy related to any drug, 547 were on statins. The fact of the matter is that once the FDA's MedWatch gets its act together and reports the true frequency of statin associated peripheral neuropathy it will be an eye-opener to doctors now blinded by lack of feedback of this nature. And these are only the ones I know about in my small piece of this statin side effect pie. The true figures are almost certainly a hundred times greater for most of these statin associated peripheral neuropathy cases are not recognized as such and are grossly under reported.

As the prescribing physicians are about to learn, this is not nearly so rare a condition as they have been led to believe by the drug company funded clinical trials. First of all, drug company supported clinical trials introduce company philosophy bias and they are done by doctors having not the slightest idea of the scope or frequency of statin drug side effects. They have never been told the truth. Sure, statin victims occasionally report to MedWatch but there it sits for what amounts to perpetual study with no significant feedback to the doctors responsible for writing the prescriptions.

c.) Permanent Myopathy

When Pfizer first introduced Lipitor to the marketplace they added a warning that rare cases of rhabdomyolysis had been reported with statin use and counseled that any patient with muscle pain or weakness in conjunction with increased CPK to 10 times the upper limit of normal had myopathy and should be treated as such. Rhabdomyolysis can be considered as a particularly aggressive type of myopathy involving inflammation of many muscle groups rather than restricted to just one area and associated with muscle cell wall breakdown.

Most of us are well aware of the 100 or so rhabdomyolysis deaths associated with use of the ill-fated Baycol. Few are aware that several hundred more rhabdomyolysis deaths have occurred since then from the other statin drugs. All reductase inhibitors can trigger this dread condition but none with the same aggressiveness as Baycol.

It should be noted that the FDA did not allow AstraZeneca the full range of dosages requested for Crestor. Permission for the highest dose was denied and Crestor remains the one statin with a rhabdomyolysis record closest to Baycol and must be watched closely, especially with its other specific renal toxicity factor.

Otherwise, all that is noted for muscles in Pfizer's adverse drug events warning to doctors is leg cramps, myasthenia and myositis. Nowhere in any drug company literature is mention made of the fact that the muscle aches, pains and weakness might become permanent. Dr. Beatrice Golomb reports that 68% of the statin myopathy patients become permanent in her series of permanent myopathy sufferers.

Several years ago I had the opportunity to talk with two astronaut friends who told me of their Lipitor experiences. In both cases Lipitor had been started by NASA physicians at the time of their routine physicals at Johnson Space Center. The reason for use of a statin then was purely because their total cholesterol value had finally exceeded the "norm." After some six to eight weeks both men told me they had to stop their Lipitor because of leg aches and pains. To their surprise the leg pain did not cease after their stopping the offending drug, instead it intensified and remained at a barely tolerable level. Never before in their busy lives had they noticed leg aches and pains. Now this condition seemed chronic. Three years had passed by the time I talked with them and both were quite bitter about their personal experiences with statins. Need I add that an experience such as this has permanent consequences on the doctor/patient relationship?

It was at about this time I noted that my repository of statin side effect reports was showing a small but growing sub-group of patients with a primary complaint being muscle aches and pains persisting for months and even years after they had stopped the offending statin. In some cases their statin had been changed from one brand to another in their doctor's futile quest to find an acceptable one before discovering that now their muscle pain problem seemed permanent despite their having stopped everything.

I can report that about a quarter of my myopathy reports are of the persistent type. Dr. Golomb's figure of 68% reflects a different population in that people seek her out for further evaluation at her office at the San Diego College of Medicine, so her additional load of difficult cases is undoubtedly the reason for her high frequency of permanent myopathy.

A permanent change in muscle physiology seems to be triggered in some people by statin use. Some of these cases seem to slowly evolve into an ALS-like picture with gradual loss of muscle mass and fasciculations. Others have the gradual addition of neuropathic symptoms with numbness to touch, pain and temperature sensations in a pattern I have come to call chronic neuromuscular degeneration and still others stay the original course of persistent muscle pain and weakness.

As to mechanism of action, just in these past few years have we learned of the role of Lrp4 in the neuromuscular junction. The substance connects agrin of the nerve ending to the muscle fiber, MuSK. Only then is acetylcholine released to effect muscle contraction. In the absence of sufficient Lrp4 this vital agrin/MuSK connection cannot occur. Since we now know that Lrp4 is a low density lipoprotein, no doubt produced by the mevalonate pathway, it is logical that failure of synthesis of sufficient Lrp4 should be considered as one of the possible mechanisms of action of statins, readily explaining chronic myopathies and, of course, even the ALS-like reactions.

We have already covered those muscle problems associated with selenoprotein inhibition by statins, creating a clinical picture much like that seen in selenium deficiency. Of the remainder, many muscle complaints regress with CoQ10 supplementation, suggesting that statin blockade of mevalonate-path CoQ10 synthesis is a major contributing problem initially, resulting in loss of cell wall integrity. The chronic cases rarely respond to CoQ10 alone and likely reflect mitochondrial mutation or inhibition of normal phosphorylation. Many of the remaining cases of myopathy reflect genetic predisposition. We are just beginning to understand the full scope of statin effects on our bodies and are only now just beginning to convey to practicing physicians what mevalonate blockade really means.

d.) Chronic Neuromuscular Degeneration

In my repository of adverse reactions associated with statin use I now have several hundred case reports of a spectrum of lingering and even slowly progressive muscle and nerve complaints apparently brought on by the use of statins. Generally these complaints consist of burning pain with tingling or numbness of the extremities associated with various aches and pains, weakness and loss of muscle size. Some victims described their muscles as unusually soft or even "mushy." Poor coordination, trouble rising from a seated position, unsteadiness and tendency to fall are also reported along with general weakness and easy fatigability. Usually these symptoms have started within a few months after statin treatment has begun but in some cases victims have been on the drug at unchanged dose for protracted periods of a year or more.

The worst feature of this condition is not only its failure to respond to the stopping of statin treatment but to the tendency to slowly progress. Many inexperienced clinicians with perhaps excessive focus on cholesterol levels have instructed patients to discontinue their present statin and substitute another, to no avail. Since all statins have the same mechanism of action—that of reductase inhibition—there is little justification to think that substituting statins will work for this subgroup of patients. Most primary care physicians will be unable to offer an explanation for the persistence of symptoms after drug cessation and will rightfully refer for specialist evaluation. Even specialists are challenged with the progressive nature of the condition, especially when workups for "all the usual suspects" turn up negative. Most of these victims wind up with such diagnoses as chronic peripheral neuropathy or chronic neuromyopathy. More for personal convenience than anything else, I have labeled this condition chronic neuromuscular degeneration because it has characteristics of both nerve and muscle pathology. And perhaps the word degeneration is appropriate because to me it suggests the continuing nature of the process.

Until a few years ago, I considered myself to be very fortunate that my personal reactions to two months of Lipitor 10mg/day in 1999 and four months of Lipitor 5mg/day in 2000 was transient global amnesia, an inability to formulate new memory with retrograde amnesia for years into the past. At least with this condition, when you finally come to your senses, you are normal with no deficits. Now that I have learned about this condition of statin associated chronic neuromuscular degeneration I realize that this has been my true underlying diagnosis, not spinal stenosis and degenerative arthritis.

With my leg pain and back pain and shrinkage of muscles in my right leg five years ago, came an unusual easy fatigability and weakness. Sure I had imaging evidence of moderate spinal stenosis and degenerative arthritis. What 70-year old male does not after a lifetime of heavy physical activity? However, on the basis of the imaging study results and my personal conviction that it was fixable surgically, I went ahead with the surgery. When I continued to fail despite my lower lumbar fusion, I went on to a second operation for complete spinal fusion with long titanium rods from my lumbar spine to lower thoracic region. Now, several frustrating years later, I find myself worse than I was before my first fusion. I am also wiser now, for with the help of my repository of reports of statin victims, belatedly, I know that my true diagnosis during this entire time has been chronic neuromuscular degeneration somehow triggered by statins. The only ones to benefit from my spine stabilizing surgery were my surgeon and the hospital.

What is the possible mechanism of action whereby a mevalonate pathway reductase inhibitor–a statin–can affect muscles and nerves in such a manner that even after stopping statins the neuromuscular condition slowly worsens? The vital functions of the mevalonate metabolic pathway include the following: 1) Cholesterol synthesis, 2) CoQ10 synthesis, 3) Dolichol synthesis 4) Normal Geranyl-geranyl phosphorylation, 5) Selenoprotein synthesis and 6) Synthesis of nuclear factor-*kappa* B.

Draeger's findings[1] support the hypothesis that statin induced cholesterol lowering per se contributes to myocyte damage and suggests further that it is the specific lipid/protein organs of the skeletal muscle itself that renders it particularly vulnerable. He did skeletal muscle biopsies from statin treated and non-statin treated patients and examined them using electron microscopy and biochemical approaches. They reported clear evidence of skeletal muscle damage in statin treated patients despite their being asymptomatic.

Caso[2] reports that "myopathy may be related in part to statin inhibition of the endogenous synthesis of coenzyme Q10, an essential co-factor for mitochondrial energy production." He found that "after a 30-day intervention study, pain severity decreased by 40% (p <0.001) and pain interference with daily activities decreased by 38% (p <0.02) in the group treated with coenzyme Q." CoQ10 has long been known to have a role both in cellular structural integrity and in mitochondrial energy production.

William Campbell,[3] in the October 2006 issue of *Muscle and Nerve,* presents a number of statin associated neuromuscular problems recently encountered by clinicians and an excellent review of the vital role of cholesterol with its extraordinary sensitivity to statin manipulation in some people. He goes on to discuss polymyositis-like cases requiring steroids that point to a pro-inflammatory effect of statins. Campbell proposes a previously unsuspected effect of statins on muscle cell lipid/protein "rafts" recently described, that results in a tendency to apoptosis (cell death and disintegration). It is these remnants of apoptosis that incite the autoimmune reaction and cause the inflammatory response. Campbell also discusses the dolichols, another vital product synthesized through the mevalonate pathway and hence inhibited by statins. Researchers now know that cholesterol and other lipids are not evenly distributed throughout a cell but exist with proteins as cholesterol "rafts" having key roles in cell signaling and all this under the direction of dolichols, giving us still another way in which statin drugs can complicate the lives of some people.

Georgirene Vladutiu[4] PhD of the Robert Guthrie Genetics Laboratory in Buffalo thinks that some patients may have a genetic susceptibility to statin use. Special genetic susceptibility may explain not only much of the statin associated rhabdomyolysis but also the curious pattern of persistent myopathy, often following only a short course of statins. Since susceptibility testing of this type is not yet available, there is no way to identify these susceptibles until the damage is done. One of these genetically determined enzymatic conditions is carnitine palmitoyl transferase (CPT) deficiency. The enzymes involved are found on different membranes of our mitochondria, those busy factories within each of our cells responsible for the production of our adenosine triphosphate (ATP) energy. Produced in each of the body's million's of cells, mitochondrial ATP is the body's sole source of energy. CPT enzymes work together with Coenzyme Q10 in the process of transport of fatty acids into our mitochondria and their ultimate conversion into fuel. Deficiency of this class of enzymes is characterized by unusual muscle pain and stiffness after exercise or work.

Mooseman and Behl[5] postulate that this type of myopathy is due to direct interference of the isopentyl step of the mevalonate pathway as a consequence of the almost inevitable statin induced fall in available selenoproteins. The substrate for this reaction, isopentenyl pyrophosphate IPP, is a direct metabolite of mevalonate. All statins inhibit this function. The resulting clinical picture of statin associated myopathy includes a non-uniform pattern of muscle aches and pains, weakness and tenderness with easy fatigability. It can vary from mild to very severe, or even be disabling. This pattern of signs and symptoms is very similar clinically and pathologically to those induced by severe selenium (selenoprotein) deficiency, supporting their hypothesis.

Of the various possibilities, I am betting on Caso's mitochondrial damage.

CHAPTER 15
Mitochondrial Mutations:
Dietary Supplements of Potential Benefit

Dietary supplements reviewed in this chapter have not been evaluated by the U.S. FDA for the possible benefits described. This information is not intended to diagnose, treat, cure or prevent disease.

Relevant to statin damage, we recently have learned much about natural causes of mitochondrial damage. Studies of chronic fatigue and other infirmities of age have pointed to the progressive loss of the ability of our mitochondria to produce high-energy molecules (ATP) for cell function. We now know that progressive damage to our mitochondria results from exposure to the so-called free radicals. These highly reactive species inevitably lead to modifications of mitochondrial lipids, proteins and DNA, known as mutations, and are a consequence of natural aging.

Ordinarily our antioxidant system is sufficient to overcome this daily oxidative stress but due to the combination of our predetermined genetic make-up, nutrition factors and exposure to disease, our anti-oxidation capacity, never 100% in its effectiveness, gradually deteriorates as we age. This allows excess build-up of so-called reactive oxygen species (ROS), the primary cause of the mitochondrial damage or mutations that accumulate as we age.

This knowledge has supported the development recently of a huge research effort directed at the use of nutritional supplements in attempting to bolster our failing metabolic and anti-oxidation systems. Every aspect of our energy equation has been studied and thousands of research studies have been done to determine possible benefit from supplementing this or that vital substance of oxidative phosphorylation and anti-oxidation pathways.

Now we find that among the many side effects of statin drug use is the same direct assault on our mitochondrial DNA and our energy equation produced by natural aging. The well-known statin side effect of coenzyme Q10 inhibition bears directly upon the effectiveness of our anti-oxidation system, leading directly to excess ROS production with its aging-like mutagenic consequences. Additionally, another well-known statin side effect, that of dolichol inhibition, results directly in failure of glycoprotein synthesis and loss of effectiveness of many of our glycoprotein based systems, such as glycohydrolases for detection and correction of DNA damage. Statin drugs cause effects on our mitichondria identical to those that accumulate with age. One might say that one side effect of statin therapy is premature aging.

My studies over the past several years have slowly revealed the various mechanisms of action of the statin drugs in the production of side effects. First I learned about statin drug inhibition of glial cell cholesterol, so vital for memory. Then, on the basis of observations of coenzyme Q10 and dolichol reductions, I learned about the inevitable mevalonate blockade by statins with resulting neuropathies, myopathies and chronic neuromuscular degeneration. And now I know why many of the statin side effects are permanent and why weakness and fatigue are such common complaints. Many statin victims say that abruptly, almost in the blink of an eye, they have become old people.

MD's, for the most part unaware of the truth because the FDA has not informed them, reassuringly say, "You have to expect these things now at your age. You are not thirty anymore." Unwittingly doctors have come close to the mark, for aging is what statins do!

Treatment of this effect of statins must involve all that nutritional researchers have learned these past few years in their quest for youth. Need I remind you that there is no traditional medical pharmaceutical treatment for the prevention and treatment of mitochondrial mutations. Everything that nutritional researchers consider useful and appropriate for fatigue and aging therapy is completely relevant for statin damage treatment. The list of substances found to be relevant to the process of oxidative phosphorylation and anti-oxidation in the human body is extensive:

Anti-oxidants found useful: Vitamin C, Vitamin E (tocotrienols and tocopherols), Coenzyme Q10, Alpha-Lipoic Acid, N-acetyl cysteine, Carotenoids, Flavonoids, Proanthocyanidins and Selenium.

Important Accessory Molecules: Vitamin B3 (niacin), Vitamin B6 (pyridoxine hydrochloride), Vitamin B12 (cyanocobalamin), Vitamin B2 (riboflavin), Folic Acid (folate), Melatonin, Magnesium, Zinc, Phosphatidylcholine and related compounds, Glyconutrients, and D-Ribose.

There is no way the average person can look at this list and formulate their personal requirements for mitochondrial repair. Even medical professionals, after a lifetime of experience, must work hard to convert these elements of metabolism and anti-oxidation into a rational plan for help. Fortunately, there have been exceptions.

Well known cardiologist, Stephen Sinatra M.D., after studying the energy equation of the heart following the introduction of statin drugs, had long been an advocate of certain supplements in his busy practice. He has advised the routine use of CoQ10, L-carnitine and magnesium for years and, more recently, has added D-ribose. He also became very selective in the use of statins. William Summers M.D. Internist, has developed a broad spectrum formulation of supplements vital for the energy needs of the body.

Although we have the technological ability to measure the various components of our electron transport, oxidative phosphorylation and *beta*-oxidative systems, the cost of doing so would be prohibitive and the only rational approach is to administer supplements on a broad spectrum basis.

I have taken on the task of selecting those thirteen that most impress me with their potential to help slow down or reverse this process of statin associated mitochondrial mutations. I will present each one without regard for relative effect and discuss my reasoning.

1.) CoQ10 – Coenzyme Q10 in blood and tissue has been shown repeatedly to be depleted following the start of statin therapy. The reason for this is now thoroughly understood – the mevalonate blockade resulting from the use of reductase inhibitors (statin drugs). Not only does mevalonate inhibition result in reduction of cholesterol synthesis, it also results inevitably in the inhibition of coenzyme Q10 synthesis, for both use the same mevalonate metabolic pathway. Never was there the slightest doubt of this in the minds of drug company pharmacists and biochemists. Not only does CoQ10 play a vital role in the energy equation whereby our mitochondria produce adenosine triphosphate (ATP) but it also has a powerful anti-oxidant role. In the absence of sufficient quantities of CoQ10 our mitochondria are exposed to the full impact of free radical damage, increasing their already high mutation rate many times over. The reason for the emphasis on CoQ10 anti-oxidation over and above other equally powerful anti-oxidants is because it already is there in our mitochondria as a major substrate in oxygen transfer. So before you consider any other choice, take CoQ10 in robust doses.

I used to say take all you can afford for there is no upper limit on this natural substance. I said that somewhat jokingly because of its cost. But the cost is coming down. I used to think 200mg daily was reasonable, and perhaps it is for prevention, but if you have symptoms, consider 600mg, even 1,000 for a therapeutic trial. Many studies of doses up to 1,500mg daily have been used in supervised studies.

2.) Vitamin C – Vitamin C, found in a variety of fruits and vegetables, is essential not only for good health, but our very survival. Without vitamin C, human beings will certainly die of scurvy, a disease characterized by bleeding gums, skin discolorations from small, ruptured blood vessels, easy bruising, joint pain, and loose and decaying teeth. Vitamin C has many essential roles in the body. Primary among these is the synthesis of collagen, which is a main structural protein in our bodies, giving support to tissues, including strengthening our blood vessels, ligaments, tendons, bones, and teeth. It is for this role that we, millions of years ago, transformed our capacity for vitamin C synthesis into that for making the highly thrombogenic Lp(a). Imagine the advantages of a molecule studded with receptors for lysine, glycine and proline, the components of collagen. The slightest tear into these collagen strands from whatever cause, must inevitably rupture one or more of these collagen threads thereby triggering the immediate clustering of Lp(a) about the damaged area, stopping blood loss. Is it any wonder that excess Lp(a) activity, this gift from our ancestors, is considered harmful in today's world, free of "tooth and claw" worries?

Vitamin C is also required for the synthesis of hormones, neurotransmitters, and other important substances needed for metabolism. In addition to these functions, vitamin C is a powerful antioxidant. It neutralizes free radicals before they have a chance to damage our cells. The importance of this anti-oxidant role of vitamin C is just being discovered. Vitamin C is arguably one of the most important antioxidants in our human physiology for its versatility and wide ranging presence.

The only argument one might have with the government's Recommended Daily Allowance (RDA) is that all the many roles of vitamin C have not been accounted for. The current RDA is adequate to prevent death or serious health issues from acute deficiency of vitamin C (e.g., scurvy). The RDA is also adequate for required collagen and hormone synthesis (the RDA is mainly based on this). But to work effectively as an antioxidant, scientists are learning that vitamin C levels need to be significantly higher in our bodies. And the debate now is over how much is needed.

According to Linus Pauling, a two-time Nobel Prize winning chemist who is noted for his research in this field, our early human ancestors probably consumed several grams per day of vitamin C from their diet. This is much higher than today's RDA for an adult man.

It was not until 1928 that vitamin C was isolated. Shortly thereafter its powerful anti-oxidant role was determined, placing vitamin C on nearly a par with CoQ10 in this function. The role of anti-oxidants in nutrition is to minimize the production of free radicals.

Free radicals have been shown to be a significant contributing factor in the development of chronic disease and cancer. Free radicals can also oxidize LDL cholesterol. As we're learning, it's not so much the LDL cholesterol that's implicated in the development of heart disease, it's that the LDL cholesterol has been "oxidized" by free radicals that is important. Free radicals can also cause DNA mutation and damage the supportive structure of our cells, which can contribute to the development of cancer and free radicals; these appear to be the essence of aging.

The Recommended Daily Allowance (RDA) of vitamin C in the past has not sufficiently considered this vital role of vitamin C in anti-oxidation and complicating everything is the fact that vitamin C is a water-soluble vitamin, which means that it is not stored in the body and must be replaced by our diet every day. The Tolerable Upper Intake Level (UL) is the maximum continual intake of a nutrient that is unlikely to cause adverse health effects in almost all people and for vitamin C has been defined to be 2g/day (2,000 mg/day). Therefore, healthy individuals have little concern of toxicity if consuming more vitamin C than specified by the RDA and 2gms, today's recommended UL, would appear to be an acceptable starting dose.

One word of caution - people who have a high risk of kidney disease or disorders of iron metabolism should avoid large doses of vitamin C (>500mg) and, as always, you should adhere to your doctor's advice.

3.) Selenium - Only in the past decade has the medical community been aware of the complex and vital role of selenium and selenoproteins in human health. Much of this gain in knowledge has come from the increasing awareness of the inhibitory effect of statin drugs on selenoprotein synthesis. As reductase inhibitors, all statin drugs inevitably block the mevalonate pathway to varying degrees because of the prevailing priority in the medical community to inhibit cholesterol synthesis. The concurrent inhibition of selenoprotein synthesis is inevitable along with inhibition of CoQ10 and dolichol as well. Many reports of myopathy and even cognitive alterations have been received where altered selenoprotein metabolism associated with statin use has been suspected.

Selenium, in certain compounds, is of fundamental importance to human health. It is an essential component of several major metabolic pathways, including thyroid hormone metabolism, anti-oxidation and immuno-defense. Ten years have elapsed since recommended dietary intakes of selenium were introduced in the UK and other European Union countries on the basis of blood glutathione peroxidase activity. I have written before on the combined value of glutathione and CoQ10 in the process of mitochondrial oxidative phosphorylation so critical to ATP energy formation. Since then, 30 new selenoproteins have been identified, of which 15 have been purified sufficiently to allow beginning clarification of their biological function but at the time of this writing we are only scratching the surface as to the many faces of selenium.

We all recognize the importance of selenium to human health but our awareness of selenium's critical role is so new we are unable at this time to deduce the long term health implications of declining selenium intakes in the elderly, recently noted. Nor can we respond to the impact of statin drugs on selenium bio-availability as millions of people are urged to take these drugs, many of them, these same elderly. The impact of all this has not been sufficiently examined at this time, yet in every direction researchers turn, new fertile avenues of exploration appear, leading to fields of ever more involved biologic interactions.

One researcher states his frustration at never finding the bottom of this cornucopia of selenoprotein research opportunities thusly: "To date, nearly all selenoproteins appear to have enzymatic activities where they likely participate in redox reactions. However, the amino acid sequences, enzymatic activities, tissue distribution of expression, and other molecular features of the different family members are extremely varied. Similarly, at the physiological level, these enzymes are involved in diverse metabolic and physiological functions ranging from antioxidant defense to fertility, muscle development and function, thyroid hormone metabolism, and immune function. Consequently, the range of pathologies associated with primary or secondary defects of selenoprotein function is enormous, with no easily definable unifying feature to tie together this disparate group of phenotypes at the pathophysiological level."

Only in the past few years has the full spectrum of selenium's role in health been revealed. Mooseman and Behl's authoritative and current review has done much to illuminate the various roles of selenoproteins in body function.[1] Much of the stimulus for this recent work has been the awareness that selenoprotein synthesis is one of the major biological pathways inhibited when statins block the mevalonate pathway. We are only just beginning to understand the full range of selenoprotein involvement but cognitive dysfunction and myopathies are already well known consequences of selenium and selenoprotein lack. Dosing selenium in proper compounds at 100mcg to 200mcg daily impresses me as being reasonable.

4.) Glyconutrients - No longer do we consider sugars as just simple fuel. The effects of these vital sugars on the resulting peptide structure being created in the endoplasmic reticulum and companion piece, the Golgi apparatus, is just short of miraculous. Statin damage is often additive to pre-existing impairment of glycolysis from aging, disease and poor nutrition. And this attachment of sugars, this glycolysis, is completely dependent on dolichol's orchestration. Throw in a statin and what do you have? – an inevitable inhibition of dolichol (roughly comparable to the degree of cholesterol inhibition). The resulting effect upon the body of this dolichol theft is completely unpredictable for this is the very center of neuropeptide synthesis (our molecules of emotion) cell identification, cell communication and immunodefense.

Dolichols may well be fully as important as CoQ10 in this unfortunate game of statin roulette that Big Pharma has placed us in and unfortunately dolichol as such is not available as a supplement. I look to glyconutrients, now increasingly available as a source of these vital sugars, as a possible way of helping the body overcome relative dolichol lack by the relative surplus of these key sugars in our cells, thereby assisting glycoprotein synthesis. This offers possible hope to thousands of statin damaged victims to help the body repair the effects of lack of dolichol availability and impaired glycolysis. I have already mentioned the importance of glycohydrolases in repair of DNA errors. This glycoprotein is vital to detecting the error, cutting out the damaged area and inserting a replacement. Anything we can do to enhance the function of glycoprotein synthesis may help offset statin damage to the mitochondria.

In contrast to drugs, the glyconutrients do nothing directly and utilized as nutrient units they are used to assemble bioactive compounds as instructed in the coding written in the genes that control cellular synthesis. Glyconutrients do not work in every individual, but they are not by their chemical nature poisons and do not damage vital organs.

5.) Lecithin – Lecithin is a phospholipid found primarily in egg yolks and soy. Of all the phospholipids, phosphatidylcholine is singularly the most important. The powerful, even miraculous, reports of extensive studies over the past several decades in the U.S. and in Europe have established a firm understanding of its relationship to aging and diseases of old age. Of the tens of thousands of molecules that make up the life of a cell, phosphatidylcholine stands apart as the major component of the membrane, the structural skin that surrounds the cell as well as the tiny organelles within it. But it is far more than an outside protective layer; it is literally the essence of life. Cellular membranes are bi-lipid layers of opposing phospholipids, lined up soldier fashion, that automatically organize themselves in a spherical shape to provide the protecting outer cover. Within this membrane sits a huge selection of ion channels and receptors from our genetic library that literally run the entire system. Some 70% of these phospholipid molecules are essential fatty acids and must be derived from diet. As with selenium, one simply cannot do justice to the importance of this substance in a single paragraph and the interested reader is referred to internet search. Suffice it to say that phosphatidylcholine is of vast importance to mitochondrial health. Lecithin is good for you. How good? Each tablespoon (7.5 grams) of lecithin granules contains about 1,700 mg of phosphatidyl choline, 1,000 mg of phosphatidyl inositol, and about 2,200 mg of essential fatty acids as linoleic acid. It also contains the valuable fish-oil-like, omega-3 linolenic acid. It is the rule, not the exception, for one or more of these valuable substances to be undersupplied by the daily diet. Take capsules or granules at fully recommended doses.

6.) Omegas 3 & 6 (essential fatty acids):

Much has recently been learned about the omegas, 3 and 6 and their usefulness, even necessity, in mitochondrial maintenance. Until very recently the emphasis was solely on omega-3, portrayed as the omega of primary importance. This concept has recently been challenged and much of the following is based on revolutionary research on PEOs (Parent Essential Oils)

There are two families of essential fatty acids: omega-3 fatty acids and omega-6 fatty acids. Both are termed "essential" because they cannot be produced by the body and must therefore be obtained from the diet. The inflammation suppression potential of the essential fatty acids (EFAs) has been found to be of great importance in arterial inflammation.

There is no longer any doubt as to the vital role of these polyunsaturated fatty acids in reducing cardiovascular disease risk. Not only has it been firmly documented to stabilize the myocardium electrically, resulting in reduced ventricular arrhythmias and sudden cardiac death, but also they have been found to have potent anti-inflammatory effects quite comparable to those of the statin drugs.

Recent studies have discovered EFA's strong anti-inflammatory effects are due to their ability to be converted into anti-inflammatory prostaglandins. What hasn't been properly reported though is that unadulterated omega-6 is the basis, technically called the substrate, for the body's most potent natural anti-inflammatory prostaglandin PGE^2 which Michael Schmidt PhD reported in his book, *Smart Fats*, as much more powerful than the omega-3 series.

Until recently, the typical western diet has evolved to be relatively high in omega-6 and relatively low in omega-3 fatty acids so that the emphasis for supplementation has been almost exclusively on omega-3. Unfortunately, due to extensive food processing required to stop the oxygen transfer so foods don't quickly turn rancid, we find that much of the ingested omega-6 has been inactive, rendered thus by food preservation, processing, storage and cooking so that our PEOs are deficient both in amount and in ratio of one to the other. Omega balance is the key to proper metabolism. Note that parent omega-3 oils are rarely used in frying or baking because they are too reactive, so essentially all of the harmful processing occurs with the parent omega-6 oils only. Nutritionists and physiologists are calling attention to this need for proper functional balance in the ratio of omega-6/omega-3 that we consume. Unfortunately, most supplemental recommendations are wrong because they don't account for the substantial amount (greater than 50%) of adulterated and therefore unavailable parent omega-6 in foods today.

Because of recent pioneering work, some physicians are beginning to use the term "parent" essential oil, stressing that our intake must focus on the parent omega-6 (linoleic acid, LA) and parent omega-3 (alpha-linolenic acid ALA) that we eat each day, not their derivatives. As I look at my bottle of omega-3, I see that it is composed mostly of the derivatives EPA (eicosapentaenoic acid) and DHA (docosahexaenoic acid) – almost nothing of the parent omega-3 which likely was flaxseed oil. And it is the same with omega-6, having derivatives GLA (gamma-linolenic acid) and CLA (conjugated linoleic acid) and nothing of the original sunflower oil, the likely parent. We then are often buying mainly the derivatives which have given pharmacological overdoses of these omega derivatives when all we need are the parents since our bodies immediately create whatever derivatives we require, reserving a very substantial amount of the parent for other vital anti-inflammatory activities as *American Journal of Clinical Nutrition*[3] made clear in their conclusions:

"Conclusions: The consumption of ALA-enriched supplements for 12 wk was sufficient to elevate erythrocyte EPA and docosapentaeoic acid content, which shows the effectiveness of ALA conversion and accretion into erythrocytes. The amounts of ALA required to obtain these effects are amounts that are easily achieved in the general population by dietary modification."

Only recently have we learned that EFAs are no longer present in sufficient quantities or proportions in our foodstuffs. One of the most significant changes has been in feeding cattle on grain, not grass like Nature intended. This has drastically altered the ratio of omega-6/omega-3 in the meats widely consumed. Similarly, eggs from present day penned, corn-fed chickens is drastically altered in ratio of omega-6/-3 from what it used to be. Adding to this has been the effect of modern food-processing. Virtually every processed product on supermarket shelves has been substantially altered, artificially, for increased shelf life. The palatability of these products is unchanged but fatty acid function, often severely curtailed, compromised and ineffective, is incorporated in each of the body's 100 trillion cells.

It is true that the ratio of omega-3 to omega-6 in the diet in the West has been falling for decades, closely paralleling the rise in heart disease during the same time period. However this has been accompanied by progressive deterioration in the quality of omega-6, especially, due to the afore-mentioned factors of food storage, processing and cooking. A newly discovered balance of omega-6 and omega-3 fatty acids is essential for proper health and we can achieve this only by supplementing our omegas together.

Decades of research has failed to show the precise mechanism by which omega-3 exerts its beneficial effect on reduction of cardiovascular disease risk. Biochemistry and physiology suggest that supplemental omega-3 intake is important but so is solving the adulterated omega-6 problem. Our most important established truth is the now thoroughly documented role of EFAs in oxygen transfer. Oxygen from the blood diffuses readily throughout the body's lipophilic unsaturated fatty acids, transferring into cellular mitochondrial membranes with ease. Both structure and function of the inner mitochondrial membrane and its four, protein/lipid respiratory chain complexes serve the need for oxygen transfer in ATP production. It reflects the perfection of evolutionary design.

We are constantly reminded in work of this kind that the problem is the proper balance of omega-6 to omega-3 in meeting the needs of the body for EFAs. Many studies have been done producing only confusion unless attempts are made to keep the omega-3 and omega-6 in proper balance.

A 2007 Harvard School of Public Health study of heart disease reported in the medical journal *Circulation* titled *"Alpha-Linolenic Acid and Risk of Nonfatal Acute Myocardial Infarction,"*[4] details some important discoveries confirming the newly discovered science of parent omega oils. Fish oil categorically failed. Here's what they stated: "Greater alpha-linolenic acid [parent omega-3] (assessed either in adipose or by questionnaire) was associated with lower risk of myocardial infarction [heart attack]. Similarly, low intakes of alpha-linolenic acid can be found in developing countries where cardiovascular disease is on the rise. Fish intake was similar in cases and controls, and the variation within each group was large.... Fish or eicosapentaenoic acid [EPA] and docosahexaenoic acid [DHA] intake at the levels found in this population did not modify the observed association.

The recommended dose of EFAs is variable, but a supplement ratio between 1:1 and 2.5:1 parent omega-6/omega-3 is probably desirable. Therefore, I take at least 2000mg to 2500mg of omega-6/-3 supplementation daily as a routine, of which 1,000 is parent omega-3 and the remainder is parent omega 6. For those wishing to meet their omega needs simply through dietary means realize it is not all that easy. For example, cooking steak, lamb or fish to well done (165°F) almost completely destroys the effectiveness of the EFAs. Sushi is fine! But it takes care to do it right. Consider supplements as your best insurance.

7.) Tocopherols, Vitamin E - Vitamin E in the form of tocopherols has generally been considered vital to the body's inflammatory response.For decades the anti-inflammatory value of tocopherols has been recognized and the public has come to regard *alpha*-tocopherol as vitamin E. Only relatively recently has the value of the previously under-recognized tocotreinol fraction of the vitamin E family been discovered. This will be reviewed in the next section. However impressive the tocotrienols are though, the original tocopherols remain an important source of anti-inflammatory activity and are an important addition to this list of potential mitochondrial maintenance supplements.

8.) Tocotrienols, Vitamin E – This is the new and, in my judgment, much improved form of vitamin E. Tocotrienols are naturally occurring members of the vitamin E family. For years they have been overshadowed by the better known tocopherols, which long have made claim to the title, vitamin E. The truth is that the vitamin E in use these past decades has been overwhelmed with tocopherols, and especially alpha-tocopherol, and was tocotrienol poor. This off-balance will need to be corrected.

Recent research has demonstrated that tocotrienol rich vitamin E deserves another look for it has much greater effectiveness as an anti-oxidant with the added ability of modest cholesterol lowering, while at the same time, raising HDL. By far the most effective and potent tocotrienol compounds are the so-called *delta* and *gamma* forms.

Tocotrienols inhibit cholesterol synthesis by a unique ability to inhibit the farnesyl-PP to farnesyl step in cholesterol synthesis, by-passing the critical mevalonate pathway completely. Scientists have long sought a way to inhibit cholesterol at a point farther along the mevalonate pathway to avoid blockade. Tocotrienols accomplish this but their real strength is not in cholesterol reduction, it is in their powerful anti-oxidant action.

Tocotrienols have shown significant tumor-inhibition activity in several studies involving breast, skin, prostate and liver cancer but it is in anti-oxidant, anti-inflammatory and neuroprotective effects that this product has demonstrated benefits far superior to tocopherols.

They inhibit oxidation of unsaturated lipids in cell membranes as well as LDL cholesterol. They also inhibit platelet aggregation and activation while at the same time reducing monocyte adhesion and macrophage recruitment, the critical elements of the inflammatory response and the method by which statins exert their benefit in reduction of atherosclerosis and cardiovascular risk. In short they appear to have the benefit of statins with none of the risk of either excess cholesterol lowering or mevalonate blockade. Preliminary research is looking positive for tocotrienols' ability to lower C-reactive protein, the best inflammatory marker at this time. For contraindications of Tocotrienols and more on biochemistry, see Chapter 12 earlier in this book under the sub-heading: *Tocotrienols, The New Vitamin E.*

9.) Magnesium - The average American consumes only 40 percent of the recommended daily allowance of magnesium. This has serious consequences, including death, in many people. Magnesium activates 76 percent of the enzymes in the body and many of these enzymes are in our mitochondrial energy equation. But the problem arises when the cell is low in magnesium, relative to calcium. Adenosine triphosphate (ATP), the "energy currency" of the cell, is magnesium dependent.

Without enough "biologically available" magnesium, the cellular calcium pump slows down. Thus, low levels of available magnesium inhibit the generation of energy. The end result is that the mitochondrion, the powerhouse of the cell and the entire body, degenerates.

10.) L-carnitine - The adult form of carnitine palmitoyltransferase (CPT) II deficiency has been labeled as the most common lipid myopathy in humans. This autosomal recessively inherited disease may be even more prevalent than generally believed due to under-recognition of the disorder. CPT II is associated with the inner mitochondrial membrane. It works together with carnitine-acylcarnitine translocase, an inner mitochondrial membrane enzyme, to facilitate the transport of lipids (fatty acids) across these membranes and into the mitochondrial matrix where they ultimately are converted to energy in the form of ATP. Individuals with this disorder may be symptom-free until they are exposed to prolonged exercise, fasting, extremes in temperature, viral infection or statin drugs. There are many people with the disorder who are completely unaware of its existence until they experience severe statin associated myopathy or rhabdomyolysis. At the other end of the spectrum there are people with mild episodic symptoms who have never had a major attack and wonder if they have a disease at all or if their symptoms of work related weakness and tiredness are "all in their mind." More than 20 different mutations have been identified in the CPT2 gene among patients with CPT II deficiency and many other mutations are yet to be identified. In the recent past, CPT II deficiency could only be diagnosed by biochemical analysis of a muscle biopsy. While this remains the best specimen for a definitive diagnosis, the enzyme's activity can also be measured in white blood cells. Bottom line is that most of this condition remains subclinical. L-carnitine and CPT play a major role in the metabolism of fatty acids by our mitochondria and also functions as an anti-oxidant.

11.) Alpha Lipoic Acid - is a vital coenzyme in our mitochondria's Krebs cycle for the production of cellular energy. In the late 1980s, researchers first identified alpha lipoic acid's powerful antioxidant role. Of special interest was the unique effect of alpha lipoic acid on other anti-oxidants. It directly recycles and extends the metabolic lifespans of vitamin C, glutathione, vitamin E and coenzyme Q10. Since Coenzyme Q10 is of major importance to our mitochondrial electron transport chain, this effect of α-lipoic acid is particularly beneficial as well as unique. Only α-lipoic acid meets the established criteria of an ideal anti-oxidant. These include ready absorption in the diet, conversion in cells and tissues into usable form, possession of a variety of antioxidant actions (including interactions with other antioxidants) in both membrane and aqueous phases, and possession of a very low toxicity. In Germany, α-lipoic acid is an approved medical treatment for peripheral neuropathy. It speeds the removal of glucose from the bloodstream, at least partly by enhancing insulin function, and it reduces insulin resistance, an underpinning of many cases of coronary heart disease and obesity.The therapeutic dose for α-lipoic acid use in Europe is 600 mg/day. In the United States, it is sold as a dietary supplement, usually as 50 mg tablets. Note that α-lipoic acid enhances the effect of other supplemental anti-oxidants.

12.) Vitamin D - Only since 2004 has its powerful role in anti-inflammation been recognized. Just before then we learned of its vital role in cancer prevention, infection suppression and other immune system function. For 50 years before that we knew only of its critical role in the regulation of calcium in our bodies and bone metabolism. I suspect there is still more yet to come from current research on vitamin D.

We are rapidly learning of the evolving roles of vitamin D in addition to bone metabolism and can even begin to postulate the reason for the development of such additional functions. The growth-arresting influence of 1,25D on cancer cells makes sense in this light because excess UVB exposure is known to damage the DNA of skin cells, which can lead them to become cancerous.

Some have also speculated that the antimicrobial response regulated by vitamin D is an adaptation that might have evolved to compensate for D's role in suppressing certain other immune system reactions—specifically, those that lead to excessive inflammation. As many of us know too well from experience, excessive UVB exposure causes sun-burned skin, which at the tissue level results in fluid buildup and inflammation. Although a limited amount of inflammation is a beneficial mechanism for wound healing and helps the immune system fight off infection, too much inflammation causes its own havoc.

Perhaps not surprisingly, then, an impressive body of work now shows that 1,25D also acts as an anti-inflammatory agent that functions by influencing immune cell interactions. For example, different subtypes of immune cells communicate by secreting factors called cytokines to initiate a particular type of immune response. Vitamin D has been shown to repress exaggerated inflammatory responses by inhibiting that cytokine cross talk. Plentiful animal research has served to corroborate this. A possible role of vitamin D in reducing the effects of excessive oxidation on our mitochondria must be considered. This immune-suppressing function of vitamin D immediately suggested a range of new therapeutic possibilities for using vitamin D or its analogues in the control of autoimmune diseases thought to be caused by overactive cytokine responses, such as autoimmune diabetes, multiple sclerosis (MS) and inflammatory bowel disease. A majority of Parkinson's disease patients were reported to have insufficient levels of vitamin D in a study from Emory University School of Medicine. They found the fraction of Parkinson's patients with vitamin D insufficiency to be 55% compared with 36% for healthy elderly individuals serving as controls.

Hundreds of studies of many different groups of varying age, sex and occupation reveal that sub-optimal levels of vitamin D appear to be the rule in this country rather than the exception. Dose: The American Academy of Pediatrics' recommended daily intake (RDI) of 200 international units (IU) for children, which many researchers have argued is suboptimal, even for rickets prevention. The RDI for adults in North America and Europe currently ranges between 200 IU and 600 IU, depending on age. After reviewing multiple studies comparing vitamin D intake and the serum concentrations of 25D produced, Harvard School of Public Health researchers and others concluded that the current RDIs are inadequate. They suggested that no less than half of U.S. adults needed to consume at least 1,000 IU of vitamin D3 daily to raise their serum 25D concentrations to the minimum healthy level of 30 ng/mL. Certainly 1,000 IU and even 2,000 IU daily seems entirely reasonable today, especially when one is symptomatic for any of the conditions mentioned above for which vitamin D may conceivably have a vital role.

13.) D-ribose - Studies indicate oral consumption of ribose leads to increased power productivity and improves the capacity of skeletal muscles to quickly recover energy levels. Our ATP levels decrease during exercise and normally take considerable time to recover. Even after days of rest, research shows that without supplementation, skeletal muscle has a limited ability to maintain peak performance during periods of repetitive high intensity exercise. High levels of cellular energy are required to keep tissues running at peak performance.

Ischemia, a condition where poor blood flow decreases the amount of oxygen reaching various tissues in the body is one result of poor cardiovascular health. When this condition occurs, ATP levels decrease by half or more. Ribose helps the heart rebuild energy by helping to generate ATP more quickly. Other studies show that following a heart attack, ribose helped ATP levels and heart function return to normal within 48 hours. Without ribose heart function was still poor after 4 weeks.

The Department of Surgery, University of Minnesota Heart Hospital studied the effects of ribose infusion in a long-term canine model of global ischemia. Global myocardial ischemia (20 min, 37°C) was produced in dogs on cardiopulmonary bypass. With reperfusion, either ribose (80 mM) in normal saline or normal saline alone was infused at 1 ml/min into the right atrium and the animals were followed for 24 hr. Ventricular biopsies were obtained through an indwelling ventricular cannula prior to ischemia, at the end of ischemia, and 4 and 24 hr post-ischemia and analyzed for adenine nucleotides and creatine phosphate levels. In both groups, myocardial ATP levels fell by at least 50% at the end of ischemia. In the ribose-treated animals, ATP levels rebounded to 85% of control by 24 hr. No significant ATP recovery occurred after 24 hr in the control dogs.

No study has better demonstrated the benefit of ribose in ATP formation. Dr. Stephen Sinatra, cardiologist and well-known health writer, strongly recommends D-ribose supplementation whenever CoQ10 is necessary, particularly with heart failure and cardiomyopathy.

Another interesting feature of this sugar supplement is that it comprises the backbone of RNA, the basis of our genetic transcription and through the removal of one hydroxyl group becomes DNA. Because of this, it is a promising element of any attempt to repair DNA damage. Additionally, once phosphorylated, ribose can become a subunit of ATP.

CHAPTER 16
My Personal Statin Experience.

When I first wrote of my personal reaction to Lipitor in *Lipitor, Thief of Memory*, I considered myself to be lucky to have had only transient amnesia episodes, for when it was over, I was back to normal, or so it seemed to me for the next several years. During this time my statin damage research gradually was revealing hundreds of cases of permanent disabling peripheral neuropathy, permanent myopathy and progressive neuro-muscular degeneration and I wondered. For suddenly, in the past few years, I have grown old, with weakness and easy fatigability and the posture and gait of an old man.

Back in 1999 when I was first started on Lipitor, I lived on the side of a mountain in Vermont. Climbing that mountain was a normal, almost daily event for me, as was cutting and splitting my own wood and doing odd jobs for my neighbors. I thrived on physical activity and work. And my exposure to Lipitor had been so minimal—a total of three and a half months at 10mg or less. My awareness of possible statin causation came to me slowly as years passed and I read report after report from statin damaged victims. Many of them exactly described my story with a gap from beginning of drug intake to onset of symptoms often measured in many years. The feeling of weakness and easy fatigability of legs and low back made me cringe at the idea of exercise. A chair became my preferred refuge. I am now a doddering old man with withered limbs; a stranger in the mirror.

If my transition to this state had been gradual, the natural result of getting old, I might have missed the relationship but to transition thusly in just a few years was clearly not normal and hundreds of other people, all statin users, were experiencing the same thing. My rheumatologist considered a possible ALS-like condition. My neurologist said he strongly suspected mitochondrial mutation secondary to statin use. Only muscle biopsy would refine this presumptive diagnosis but he had been seeing this syndrome for several years now and strongly suspected a statin causation. There is no treatment. This ALS-like condition is slowly progressive and eventually disabling.

I have now joined the ranks of hundreds of other people whose physiologic function has been seriously compromised by statins. Cases are accumulating, more rapidly now that much higher dosing is routinely used.

What about this presumptive mitochondrial mutation etiology? Does this have merit? The existence in our cells of what could be called an alien genome, our mitochondrial organelles, introduces an unusual twist of biology in our inheritance patterns.

Mitochondria are organelles that provide most of the energy our cells need for the work they do. It is in the mitochondria where CoQ10 and the reduced forms of niacin and riboflavin enter into that ingenious process of moving electrons from hydrogen molecules to one side of a mitochondrial leaf while storing the remaining protons on the other side creating an energy gradient—the magic energy resource of every cell in our bodies. It is here that oxidative phosphorylation takes place to create ATP.

Most biologists now believe that these structures evolved from micro-organisms that established symbiotic relationships with the ancestors of animal cells very early in the history of life on this planet. Survival advantage explains how it has come to be that mitochondria contain their own DNA that codes for 13 of their proteins along with RNA that specifically helps express mitochondrial information.

As with any form of DNA, mitochondrial DNA (mtDNA) sequences are susceptible to mutation. In fact, there is evidence that mitochondrial sequences may mutate at rates 3 to 5 times greater than nuclear sequences. This may be because of the front-line position of these tiny warriors in their battle to utilize oxygen without themselves being oxidized. Constantly at risk they ordinarily are well supplied with anti-oxidants.

Enter statin drugs that, while inhibiting cholesterol synthesis, halve our CoQ10 in just a few weeks through the inevitable process of mevalonate blockade. Gone is half the fuel (oxygen) of our mitochondrial engines and gone is half of one of our most important anti-oxidants, with the job of inactivation of free radicals. Abruptly our mutation rate increases at the same time our mitochondrial engines are running low on fuel. Is this something to consider as a cause of statin-altered physiology? Of course it is.

The consequences of mitochondrial mutations, however, may be very different from those that occur in nuclear DNA. First, each cell in our bodies contains about 100,000 mitochondria, each of which has 2 to 10 copies of its genome. The effect a mutation in mtDNA will have on a cell's function will therefore depend on the number of mutant organelles in a cell compared to the number of normal, or "wild type" present.

When cells divide, their mitochondria independently replicate and then distribute DNA randomly into daughter cells. This leads to variable expressions within and among tissues ranging from non-viable cells (hence death of some tissue cells) dysfunctional energy generation in others and to subthreshold changes (i.e. "silent" mutations) in others that do not affect overall cell function. What this means is that mitochondrial mutations may be variable in their clinical presentation, depending on their timing and prevalence.

Statin associated chronic neuropathy and chronic progressive myopathy may well be examples of this process in action. It seems likely that a side effect of statin drugs in some people is to trigger just this process – mitochondrial mutations of sufficient frequency and severity to express as a chronic, even progressive condition. Indeed, it is known that accumulating mitochondrial mutations contribute significantly to aging. This appears to be what we are seeing in many statin victims - thousands of cases of permanent muscle wasting, weakness and neuropathies seen usually only in advanced age. And think of the number of cases that successfully masquerade as aging and thereby escape detection.

Variability of expression may well explain why some people seem extraordinarily sensitive, showing symptoms early, while others show no apparent effect but may well be victims of the low-grade, accelerated aging type of presentation, taking years to become evident. This may also help to explain why some people may be on a statin at an unchanged dose for years before abruptly manifesting symptoms.

At the present time there is no way to prove statin etiology, just the incredible numbers that occur shortly after statins are started. And no, it does not go away when statins are stopped. There are no markers, no tumor mass, no blood level of a substance, no measurement that shouts "statins" loud enough to be heard, only thousands upon thousands of victims. And one last observation – many of these victims have been heralded by cognitive dysfunction.

I finally had to stop my daily walks, a lifelong habit. Muscles in my legs and low back it seemed could not be rehabilitated. I had just so many remaining functional muscle fibers and finally I reached the point that just standing for a few minutes was all I could do.

I could follow my wife around with a grocery cart reasonably well, but without it I would break into a cold sweat and look for a chair. My talks were no longer on my feet before a chart or blackboard. I had to sit down just like everyone else and it worked well. Before the diagnosis was made I used to wonder why I was drenched in sweat at the end of my talks. Never occurred to me it might be ALS and that I was close to exhaustion.

I have never been really exhausted before. My neurologist and I are both convinced the mechanism of action must be mitochondrial mutations. After all that's what statins do, they wipe out CoQ10 and glutathione, the primary anti-oxidant defense against free radical damage and mitochondrial mutation.

In addition to peripheral neuropathy, statin use in my case had somehow triggered a primary lateral sclerosis type of response (currently under neurological and genetic investigation) suggesting two completely different forms of statin neurological damage (nerve fiber versus neuronal.)

As to my progressive muscle weakness I had to give up walking without assistance completely as being counter-productive. On the positive side I found a three wheel walker device which transfers weight bearing to my arms and shoulders so now I am walking again with much greater stability and co-ordination.

March 2009 Update

Three months had passed during which time I knew I had become a symbol of persistence to many others in this retirement community as I passed their homes each morning dutifully pushing my walker. Then to their surprise one morning I briskly walked my path using only a lightweight walking stick. My surprise was just as great as theirs for I had no idea my response to my new supplement plan would be so impressive. One month earlier I had started my new regimen of taking all of the supplements I had deemed essential to mitochondrial maintenance.

One thing my research had shown me was that of the many supplements that have been tested by various researchers studying mitochondrial health over the past decade, twelve clearly stood out. I know this can be argued indefinitely but from my perspective as a reasonably well-trained and well-informed MD, these twelve seem to be critical.

I had tried robust doses of CoQ10 both with and without selenium for a time, and glyconutrients and lecithin for half a year while participating in a study of their combined effectiveness on peripheral neuropathy with no significant effect on the process that was robbing me of strength and stability and turning my muscles to jelly, but I had never tried all thirteen supplements together. Never for a moment did I think I could need all thirteen critical supplements simultaneously, but how else to tell my need other than all at the same time?

I also convinced myself that ultimate dosage of each was not critical as long as some was being taken in. I completely understand that this can be grossly underdone and judgment was important. I also made once daily dosing of critical importance to me. In my conservative and traditional world, if there is anything worse than opening 13 supplement bottles daily, it was having to do it twice a day. I next mandated that all supplements requiring dissolving in liquid be done at the same time for convenience sake. The rationale for use and dosage of each are discussed in the mitochondrial mutations chapter. Everyone is different and everyone's needs are different.

At the end of one week I was seeing improvement. By the middle of the fourth week I ventured forth with my walking stick (for stability) and surprised my neighbors and that's where I am at present. I am highly motivated, perhaps more than most. I keep telling myself this is all placebo effect, knowing full well that this can be very powerful. But even my wife remarks on the new muscular look of my thighs and there seems no disputing my new energy. March 2nd 2009 was my 78th birthday and my vision of an imminent wheelchair existence has been replaced by hope of active life yet.

As a word of caution, my new freedom led me on a two-mile walk through a nearby abandoned orange grove where I stumbled and almost fell while crossing a drainage ditch. I pulled some muscle fibers in my upper back while I clung for support on my walking stick. Might have been better if I had fallen but please do not take on too much too soon. Your body is never the same as it used to be.

Traditional medicine has nothing to offer. Nutritional supplements seem to be our only hope at present, using the full range known to be vital for mitochondrial function. CoQ10 is vital in prevention of statin damage but once the damage is done, all the CoQ10 in the world cannot by itself repair mitochondrial damage. The possibility of repair, it seems, can currently only come from the broad battery of nutritional supplements I cover in this book.

July 2010 Update

Another year has passed and it is again time to tell you where I am on my path through life. It is interesting that you will not find my true diagnosis in the records of my annual astronaut physicals at Johnson Space Center, nor in the office records of my neurologist, or rheumatologist, or family doctor at my VA clinic.

I naturally have told each of them that a statin associated ALS-like degeneration is the best fit diagnosis yet nothing gets written down on my record. All the reasonable tests have been done and all are uninformative. All the doctors remain clearly skeptical as we "wrap up" the session. I am playing the role of doctor when I talk with them. I am not going to deny this for no one yet has my experience. I have daily email exposure to some of the many thousands of other cases.

My doctors know nothing about this subject of mitochondrial damage and the role of CoQ10. I cannot get through to them. They are unable to accept this extraordinary diagnosis yet it is staring them in the face and they can give no other best fit diagnosis. Certain tissues of my body are failing, slowly but surely.

Five years ago I can remember feeling fortunate that my only consequence of the bite of statins had been entirely cognitive in nature. Then slowly I realized that my progressive muscle weakness and pain and incoordination was this new thing of mitochondrial damage to my entire body.

I was receiving excess oxidative damage to mitochondrial DNA. Imagine the burden of progressive failure of various tissues as the mutations pile up. This is the principle mechanism for muscle, nerve, heart and organ damage. Cholesterol inhibition is principle in memory failure but CoQ10 inhibition is principle in most of these other types of damage. In my opinion I had been hit by both.

Now I have had to give up on recreational walking for it is counterproductive. I have just been admitted to a hydrotherapy class where they will teach me aquatic measures for muscle maintenance that do not overly strain me. A light-weight walker suffices to get most places when a cane will not. All advice has been to stay away from a wheelchair because it is one-way only.

This all stirs memories of my role in space medicine, those of developing countermeasures for zero gravity deconditioning. That astronauts on the space station must use my cursed countermeasures for two hours each day date back to my research from fifty years ago. And now I am working with a group studying the use of water immersion to bring space station astronauts back like a baby in a womb. Somehow this seems all tied together.

March 2011 Update

Last week was my 80th birthday and after four years of a progressive downhill course, I am getting stronger. Once again my muscles feel like muscles instead of soft dough. With the aid of my walker, I am back to walking slightly over one mile each day with no problems. I no longer feel that walking is counterproductive. I do not ache after walking as I did before and now when I return from walking I look forward to going out again.

My new family doctor is a gem, expertly balancing her needs with mine. She has put me on aggressive pain management so my aches and pains that seemed to be wearing me down no longer rule my life. Her water exercises kept me going six months ago when my physical capacity seemed at a minimum and walking definitely was counterproductive but then four months ago I felt better and went back to walking. She put me on depo-testosterone shots monthly to help muscle development.

My supplements this past six months have been CoQ10 400mg with liberal doses of tocotrienol (vitamin E), vitamin D and vitamin C and PQQ, a new anti-oxidant mitochondrial enhancer type of thing. I don't know what to say about PQQ except the promo made a great deal of sense. Promos are supposed to do that! Bottom line, I needed a straw to hang onto. So basically I am doing anti-oxidants, pain management and testosterone shots. I have one more factor that possibly has made a contribution - that is the process of Earthing. Cardiologist Steven Sinatra introduced me to Earthing and it made sense immediately. I started grounding myself with use of a special grounding sheet in my bed just about six months ago. The mechanism of action of grounding appears to be that of neutralizing the positive ions of any inflammatory process with mother nature's free negative electrons. I had to assume my statin associated condition was associated with the usual inflammatory buildup of positive ions. Neutralizing this positive buildup with negative ions by grounding my bed and walking barefoot to maximize the entry of negative ions through the body seemed a reasonable course of action since nothing else was working.

By walking barefoot I have acquired no small number of comments from other seniors in this ultra conservative housing area. One in particular I will share with you. On this particular day I was wearing flowered casual pants while walking barefooted and an alert neighbor called my wife to warn her that I was out there walking about and "Was I all right?" We still are laughing over that one. I suppose the caller had read my book about my two episodes of statin associated transient amnesia and thought I might be having my third. I do not go out of my way to entertain my neighbors. This just happened and come to think of it you do not see many seniors in my area walking barefoot. Even at the beach they are quite apt to wear both shoes and socks.

I have to stress that my muscle aches and pains have been with me for a long time, primarily involving upper legs and lower back. Never did I think the muscle pain was caused by exercise. My original symptoms were pain and growing weakness whether I exercised or not. This is why my need for pain management. It has helped to keep me functional when my only alternative was to be an achy couch-potato. I seemed to have crossed a threshold of regaining mitochondrial function starting first with muscles.

The pain possibly is neuropathic in origin and generally expected to be resistant to treatment.

I interpret this to mean my myopathy seems to be improving while any neuropathy is lagging behind, or may never improve. I have an impression the testosterone has helped but who knows? I have to add that my testosterone level was barely detectable. I did not recall my sexual history as all that bad but who knows what it might have been?

I still focus on mitochondrial damage as the cause and have to assume that mitochondrial genesis has occurred to account for my improvement. It all fits well with my understanding of the physiology involved. If this information is of help or gives hope to others out there I will feel amply rewarded.

July 2012 Update

There has been no change in my physical abilities from a year ago, but from the moment my doctor put me on pain management I have been a new man. The constant pain in my low back and legs has gone. I have been able to do more and be a better person. And because I feel better, I think clearer and write better. I think I may have some minimal amount of cognitive loss in that I need a bit more time to find just the right word or phrase during public speaking, but overall I feel mentally sharp.

My wife tells me I am more understandable now because my talking was much too rapid previously. Looking back I think I converse better in second gear. It allows me more time for eye contact and the natural body mannerisms so important to effective communication. This is not apparent in my writing which is as good as it ever was.

There are other pluses of aggressive pain management. I am now much more able to be involved in other projects. In the past year I have been the principle investigator in the making of a motivational video aimed at high school drop-outs and military recruitment. Additionally I am giving medical support to the honor flight program, reviewing each World War II veteran and their medical records, helping to give them their long deserved day of recognition in Washington D.C. Much more challenging has been my work with USAF flight surgeons researching the cause for the recent cognitive incidents among pilots flying F-22 Raptor aircraft.

In the past year I have acquired a Kindle® e-book reader which has made acquiring books and reading much easier and more pleasurable. I am involved in a couple of e-book projects myself along with the continuation of my writing for spacedoc.com. As for dietary supplements, I concentrate on CoQ10 these days as that is the supplement I believe that is truly of benefit to those of us damaged by statins.

CHAPTER 17
Conclusion

My purpose in the choice of the book title "*The Statin Damage Crisis*" is to draw attention to the thousands of statin damaged people who have written to me about their disabling neuropathies, myopathies and a variety of neurodegenerative conditions such as ALS and Parkinsonism associated with statin use.

But the crisis is far more than this, for with the multi-billion dollar statin drug industry, physicians are rapidly losing the confidence of their patients. The so-called doctor/patient bond has never been stretched so thin.

Denying statin causality, despite obvious highly suggestive temporal relationship and often despite the drug company warnings on the package inserts, has caused much grief. The use of statin drugs in diabetics despite drug company warnings of increased peripheral neuropathy is but one example of medicine gone wrong. Why, I ask myself, do physicians push statin drugs to diabetics when the medical literature clearly states that statin treatment is associated with a sixteen times greater risk of peripheral neuropathy.

The thousands of complaints from patients suffering from aches and pains, fatigue and weakness, casually dismissed as, "You've got to expect this now that you are over fifty" is another very common example of medicine gone wrong. When did doctors stop listening to their patients?

Many doctors are so out of touch with the reality of statin side effects they cannot counsel rationally. They know only what was told to them 15 years ago, "Statins may cause a few aches and pains or liver irritation that goes away when the dose is lowered." That is all they know.

Of the thousands of post-marketing MedWatch Adverse Drug Reactions (ADRs) they largely know nothing. I have personally documented that thousands of amnesia episodes, reported via MedWatch to the FDA, remain unreported to the medical community and the average doctor is shocked into disbelief when told the truth. This is a major crisis.

Another crisis is the policy of the insurance industry to use cholesterol levels as a reason to either deny health care coverage or life insurance coverage, or to extract higher premiums. Some employers even require cholesterol levels to be below a certain number as a condition of employment. Then there is the crisis of patients being forced into taking a statin because not to do so would result in being labeled as non-compliant and facing the prospect of having to find a new doctor. This outmoded concept is based on misinterpreted Framingham data of 40 years ago and cholesterol numbers are increasingly being dismissed as a cardiovascular disease risk factor. Cholesterol level appears irrelevant to the process of atherosclerosis for most people.

Two generations of physicians have been brainwashed with the cholesterol concept of heart attack risk championed by Ancel Keys and his manipulated data. Statin drugs apparently work not by cholesterol reduction but by anti-inflammation. Only relatively recently have we known this. The wheels grind slowly in these agencies and returning truth and reason to these large administrative structures will take much time.

Another crisis, a crisis of confidence, exists for many physicians who follow cholesterol lowering guidelines yet are stunned to find out that most of the people who write these guidelines are in the direct employ of the drug companies. Which is the greater statin damage crisis, the physician who prescribed the statin drug in ignorance of potential side effects, or the physician who prescribes the statin drug with full awareness of the potential for consequences?

But the most important crisis is that of thousands of people disabled by statin associated neuro-muscular problems while thousands of physicians still remain unaware that statins can do this. The statins strike me as being catastrophic in their potential for adversely affecting the human body. It seems like another thalidomide in the making. Imagine, a drug capable not only of subtly allowing excessive oxidation and DNA damage to our mitochondria by inhibiting CoQ10 but also interfering with the daily process of DNA error correction taking place continuously to our mitochondria by simultaneously inhibiting our dolichols. To most clinicians this is meaningless. It was not taught in medical school and most have been much too busy to stay abreast of all that science. When I first read of this in my research it seemed far too complicated for me to understand. But the principles of this knowledge are very understandable. CoQ10, co-existing as it is in our mitochondria, plays a vital role in preventing excessive oxidation. In so doing it minimizes the formation of the so-called reactive oxygen species (ROS) flashing through our lipid and protein molecules, adding a methyl group here and knocking off another there resulting in completely alien effects if not corrected. And imagine, if you will, a dolichol orchestrated system of specific glycoproteins existing for the sole purpose of correcting this daily load of DNA errors. Statins decrease the bioavailability of both CoQ10 and dolichols. What more do you need to know to be suspicious that mitochondrial mutations are slowly accumulating, robbing us of our important last years?

And this entire black thing is masquerading as premature senility. Is it any wonder doctors, when hearing these patient complaints of tiredness, weakness, wobbly-kneed with burning pain and numbness, poor coordination and terrible memory, respond with a predictable, "You are over fifty now and have to expect these kinds of things." The various processes statins initiate take years to develop. So far the medical community is comfortable with blaming God for these premature disabilities and deaths and turns a deaf ear to these complaints. And I cannot yet prove a thing.

Duane Graveline M.D., M.P.H.
Former USAF Flight Surgeon
Former NASA Astronaut
Retired Family Doctor
For more information on Statin Drugs and their Side Effects, visit: **www.spacedoc.com**

Appendix A

FDA Expands List of Statin Precautions

On 28th February 2012, the U.S. Food and Drug Administration (FDA) released important new safety information on cholesterol-lowering medications—statins.

Reports of Memory Loss

FDA has been investigating reports of cognitive impairment from statin use for several years. The agency has reviewed databases that record reports of bad reactions to drugs and statin clinical trials that included assessments of cognitive function.

"The reports about memory loss, forgetfulness and confusion span all statin products and all age groups." FDA spokesperson Egan said. "These experiences are rare but those affected often report feeling "fuzzy" or unfocused in their thinking. In general, the symptoms were not serious and were reversible within a few weeks after the patient stopped using the statin." Some people affected in this way had been taking the medicine for a day; others had been taking it for years. What should patients do if they fear that statin use could be clouding their thinking? "Talk to your health care professional," Egan said. "Don't stop taking the medication; the consequences to your heart could be far greater."

The Risk of Diabetes

Diabetes occurs because of defects in the body's ability to produce or use insulin—a hormone needed to convert food into energy. If the pancreas doesn't make enough insulin or if cells do not respond appropriately to insulin, blood sugar levels in the blood get too high, which can lead to serious health problems.

A small increased risk of raised blood sugar levels and the development of Type 2 diabetes have been reported with the use of statins, according to FDA. "Clearly we think that the heart benefit of statins outweighs this small increased risk," said Egan. "But what this means for patients taking statins and the health care professionals prescribing them is that blood-sugar levels may need to be assessed after instituting statin therapy," said Egan.

The Potential for Muscle Damage

Some drugs interact with statins in a way that increases the risk of muscle injury called myopathy, characterized by unexplained muscle weakness or pain. Egan explained that some new drugs are broken down (metabolized) through the same pathways in the body that statins follow. This increases both the amount of statin in the blood and the risk of muscle injury.

FDA is revising the drug label for lovastatin to clarify the risk of myopathy. The label will reflect what drugs should not be taken at the same time, and the maximum lovastatin dose if it is not possible to avoid use of those other drugs. Patients and health care professionals should report negative side effects from statin use to FDA's MedWatch Adverse Event Reporting Program.

The issue of muscle damage has undergone some major changes from when statins first were introduced. At the original time of marketing in 1996, FDA advised that the rate of myopathy was 2% Then in 2008 we learned that 20-24% of Europeans and North Americans were carriers for the so-called statin damage gene. Now in 2012 the myopathy damage incidence rate has become 25% due to this new interaction between lovastatin with other biochemicals. When tens of millions of people are on statins, 25% suddenly has become a lot of myopathy especially when Dr. Beatrice Golomb, Director of the statin study at San Diego College of Medicine, has shown that in 68% of these people the myopathy will be permanent. It will not go away upon stopping the statin.

FDA will be changing the drug labels of popular statin products to reflect these new concerns—these labels are not the sticker attached to a prescription drug bottle, but the package insert with details about a prescription medication, including side effects.

The statins affected include:
- Altoprev (lovastatin extended-release)
- Crestor (rosuvastatin)
- Lescol (fluvastatin)
- Lipitor (atorvastatin)
- Livalo (pitavastatin)
- Mevacor (lovastatin)
- Pravachol (pravastatin)
- Zocor (simvastatin)

Appendix B.

Causes of Statin Side Effects

Statins act by inhibiting HMG-CoA reductase.

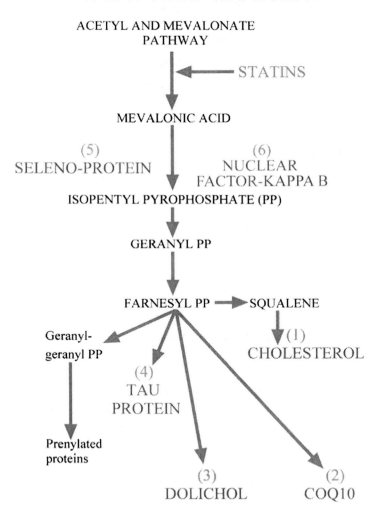

THE CAUSE OF STATIN SIDE EFFECTS

ACETYL AND MEVALONATE PATHWAY

◄— STATINS

MEVALONIC ACID

(5) SELENO-PROTEIN

(6) NUCLEAR FACTOR-KAPPA B

ISOPENTYL PYROPHOSPHATE (PP)

GERANYL PP

FARNESYL PP → SQUALENE

Geranyl-geranyl PP

(1) CHOLESTEROL

(4) TAU PROTEIN

Prenylated proteins

(3) DOLICHOL

(2) COQ10

© by Duane Graveline MD • www.spacedoc.com

All metabolic functions further down the pathway are consequently affected.

Acetyl and Mevalonate Pathway
1.) Cholesterol Inhibition
Not only is glial cell cholesterol synthesis in our brains vital for memory function and cognition, cholesterol also is the substrate for our most important hormones: aldosterone, cortisone, estrogen, progesterone and testosterone as well as the quasi-hormone, vitamin D (calcitriol). Cholesterol's vital role in membrane structure and function and lipid raft formation, makes it of critical importance in cell identification, cell communication and immunodefense.

Glial Cell Inhibition Potential Side Effects:
Amnesia
Forgetfulness
Confusion
Disorientation
Increased Senility
Hormone Lack Potential Side Effects:
Loss of Libido (sexual desire)
Erectile Dysfunction (ED)
Osteoporosis
Hair Loss

2.) CoQ10 (Ubiquinone) Inhibition
Coenzyme Q10 (CoQ10) is important for structural integrity of cells, anti-oxidation and, as part of the mitochondria, the production of Adenosine Triphosphate (ATP) energy. Part of its extreme importance in anti-oxidation is because of its location within the mitochondria, protecting the delicate components of the mitochondria from excess oxidative change and mutation.
Lack of Energy Potential Side Effects:
Chronic Fatigue Syndrome
Congestive Heart Failure
Fluid Retention
Shortness of Breath

Loss of Cell Wall Integrity Potential Side Effects:
Hepatitis
Pancreatitis
Myopathy (muscle pain and weakness, cramps)
Peripheral Neuropathy (numbness, tingling or burning
sensations particularly in hands and feet)
Rhabdomyolysis (rapid breakdown of skeletal muscle tissue)

Excessive Oxidation Potential Side Effects:
Mitochondrial Damage
Permanent Neuropathy
Permanent Myopathy
Neurodegeneration

3.) Dolichol Inhibition
Dolichols are vital to the process of glycoprotein formation in
the endoplasmic reticula of cells. In this capacity it is critical
to the formation of the glycoproteins involved in
neuropeptides, cell identification, cell messaging and
immunodefense. Reduced bioavailability of dolichols can
affect every cellular process in the body.

Neuropeptide Dysfunction Potential Side Effects:
Aggressiveness
Hostility
Irritability
Road Rage
Homicidal Behavior
Depression
Suicide

Altered Glycoprotein Synthesis Potential Side Effects:
Impairment of DNA error correction
Dysfunction of almost any cellular process
Altered cell identification
Altered cell messaging
Altered immunodefense

4.) Tau Protein Synthesis

When normal phosphorylation is interfered with by mevalonate blockade, our cells increase the production of *Tau* protein. *Tau* is the protein substance of the neurofibrilatory tangles common to Alzheimers and other neurodegenerative diseases.

Neuro-Degenerative Diseases Include:

Parkinson's Disease
Alzheimer's Disease
Amyotrophic Lateral Sclerosis (ALS)
Primary Lateral Sclerosis (PLS)
Multiple Sclerosis (MS)
Multiple System Atrophy (MSA)
Frontal Lobe Dementia

5.) Selenoprotein

Only recently discovered were selenoproteins and the effect of statin blockade of the mevalonate pathway on their role in human physiology. Deficiency of selenoproteins has been proven to result in various types of myopathies formerly seen only in areas known to be deficient in this trace element. Additionally cognitive dysfunction is known to be associated with selenium lack.

6.) Nuclear Factor - *kappa* B (NF-kB)

The benefit of statin drugs in cardiovascular disease control is in their ability to inhibit this vital transcriptase. The entire anti-inflammatory and immunomodulatory effect of statins is mediated by statin inhibition of nuclear factor-*kappa B*. Improvement in atherosclerosis results from the inhibition of the key inflammatory elements: smooth muscle migration. lymphocyte adhesion, macrophage attraction and platelet activation associated with inhibition of NF-kB. The immunodefense system is also keyed to NF-kB, explaining the changing patterns of certain infections and cancers. The rise in cancers of all kinds secondary to statin use is of major concern.

REFERENCES

CHAPTER 1 – How Statin Drugs Work

1. Brousseau ME, Schaefer, EJ, Structure and mechanism of action of HMG-CoA reductase inhibitors in *HMG-CoA Reductase Inhibitors*,Schmitz, G., Torzewski, M, Eds. Basel, Schweiz, Birkhauser, 2002.

2. Shovman O and others. Anti-inflammatory and immunomodulatory properties of statins. *Immunol Res* 25(3): 272-85, 2002

3. Masato E and others. Statin prevents tissue factor expression in human endothelial cells. *Circulation* 105:1756, 2002

4. Chen F and others. New insights into the role of nuclear factor kB in cell growth metabolism. *American Journal of Pathology* 159:387-397,2001

5. Hilgendorff A and others. Statins differ in their ability to block NF-kB activation in human blood monocytes. *International Journal of Clinical Pharmacology and Therapeutics* 41(9): 397-401, 2003

6. Karin M, Delhase M. The 1 *kappa B* kinase and NF-*kappa B*: key elements of proinflammatory signaling. *Semin Immunol* 12(1): 85-98, 2000

7. Tato CM and Hunter CM. Host-pathogen interactions: subversion and utilization of the NF-kB pathway during infection. *Infection and Immunity* 70(7): 3311-3317, 2002

8. Raggatt LJ, Partridge NC. HMG-CoA reductase inhibitors as immunomodulators: potential use in transplant rejection. *Drugs* 62(15):2185-91, 2002.

9. Kwak B and others. Statins as a newly recognized type immunomodulator. *Nature Medicine* 6:1399-1402, 2000

10. Leung BP and others. A novel anti-inflammatory role for simvastatin in inflammatory arthritis. *J Immunol* 170(3): 1524-30, 2003

11. Palinski W. Immunomodulation: A new role for statins? *Nature Medicine* 6:1311-1 312, 2000

12. Ely JTA, Krone CA. A brief update on ubiquinone (Coenzyme Q10). *J*

Orthomol Med 15(2): 63-8, 2000
13. Ely JTA, Krone CA. Urgent update on ubiquinone (Coenzyme Q10). (www.faculty.washington.edu/ely/turnover.html), 2000
14. Langsjoen P, Langsjoen E. Statin associated congestive heart failure. *Proceedings of Weston-Price Foundation Meeting,* Spring, 2003.
15. Langsjoen P, Langsjoen A. Coenzyme Q10 In cardiovascular disease with emphasis on heart failure and myocardial ischemia. *Asia Pacific Heart Journal* 7(3): 160-168, 1998.
16. Gaist D and others. Statins and the risk of polyneuropathy: A case control study. *Neurology* 58: 1333-1337, 2002.
17. Sparks S. Written personal communication. 8 August, 2003.
18. Golomb B and others. Amnesia in association with statin drug use. *UCSD statin research study* (under review) 2002.
19 Schwartz G and others. Effects of atorvastatin on early recurrent ischemic events in acute coronary syndromes. *Journal of the American Medical Association* 285 (13): 1711-1717. 2002
20. Sever PS and others. Prevention of Coronary and Stoke Events With Atorvastatin In Hypertensive Patients Who Have Average Or Lower-Than Average Cholesterol Concentrations in the Anglo-Scandinavian Cardiac Outcomes Trial. *Lancet* 361: 1149-1158, 2003
21. The ALLHAT Officers and Coordinators For the ALLHAT Collaborative Research Group. Major Outcomes In Moderately Hypercholesterolemic, Hypertensive Patients Randomized to Pravastatin vs. Usual Care: The Antihypertensive and Lipid Lowering Treatment To Prevent Heart Attack Trial. *Journal of the American Medical Association* 288: 2998-3007, 2002.
22. Collins R and others Heart Protection Study of Cholesterol Lowering With Simvastatin in 5963 People With Diabetes *Lancet* 361: 2005-2016, 2003

23. Ravnskov U. *The Cholesterol Myths*, New Trends Publishing, 2000.
24. Rosch P. Postdating drug side effects. *Proceedings of the Weston Price Foundation Meeting,* Spring 2003
25. Matsuzaki M and others. Large scale cohort study of the relationship between serum cholesterol concentration and coronary events with low-dose simvastatin therapy in Japanese patients with hypercholesterolemia. *Circ J* 66:1087-1095, 2002
26. Pfrieger F. Brain researcher discovers bright side of ill-famed molecule. *Science*, 9 November, 2001.
27. Muldoon MF and others. Effects of lovastatin on cognitive function and psychological wellbeing. *Am J Med* 2000 May: 108(7) 538-460
28. FAA headquarters, personal communication.

CHAPTER 3- Statins and Brain Cholesterol
1. Pfrieger F. Brain researcher discovers bright side of ill-famed molecule. *Science*, 9 November, 2001 .
2. Pfrieger, F. ibid.
3. Muldoon MF and others. Effects of lovastatin on cognitive function and psychological well-being. *Am J Med* 2000 May: 108(7) 538-460.........
4. Hodges JR, Warlow CP. The etiology of transient global amnesia: A case-control study of 114 cases with prospective follow-up. *Brain* 113: 639-657, 1990.
5. Wagstaff L and others. Statin associated memory loss: analysis of 60 case reports and review of the literature. *Pharmacotherapy* 23(7): 871-880, 2003.

CHAPTER 4 – Statins and CoQ10
1. Ely JTA, Krone CA. A brief update on ubiquinone (Coenzyme Q10*). J Orthomol Med* 15(2): 63-8, 2000
2. Ely JTA, Krone CA. Urgent update on ubiquinone (Coenzyme Q10).
(www.faculty.washington.edu/ely/turnover.html), 2000.

3. Langsjoen P, Langsjoen E. Statin associated congestive heart failure. *Proceedings of Weston-Price Foundation Meeting, Spring, 2003.*
4. Langsjoen P, Langsjoen A. Coenzyme Q10 In cardiovascular disease with emphasis on heart failure and myocardial ischemia. *Asia Pacific Heart Journal 7(3): 160-168, 1998.*
5.Gaist D and others. Statins and the risk of polyneuropathy: A case control study. *Neurology 58: 1333-1337, 2002.*
6. Phillip PS and others. Statin-associated myopathy with normal creatine kinase levels. *Ann Int Med* 137(7): 581-85, 2002
7. Ely JTA, Krone CA. A brief update on ubiquinone (Coenzyme Q10). *J Orthomol Med* 15(2): 63-8, 2000.
8. Wallace DC. Mitochondrial DNA in aging and disease. *Sci Amer 40-7.*
9. Ibid.
10. Wolfe S. Public citizen petitions FDA to warn doctors, patients about cholesterol drugs, 20 August, 2001
11. Whitaker J. Citizens' petition filed with FDA to include coenzyme Q10 use recommendation in all statin drug labeling. *Life Extension Magazine,* May 23, 2002

CHAPTER 5 – Statins and Dolichols

1. Griffiths G, Simons K. The Trans-Golgi Network: Sorting at the Exit Side of the Golgi Complex, *Science* 243: 438-442, 1986.
2. Pert C. *Molecules of Emotion*, Scribner, New York, 1997
3. Lambrecht BN. Immunologists getting nervous: neuropeptides, dendritic cells and T cell activation. *Respiratory Research* 2: 133-38, 2001
4. Norris JF and others. Neurosecretion: Retrospectives and Perspectives. HW Korf and KH Usadel, Eds. Springer, Berlin, 71-85,1997
5. Hokfelt T and others. General Overview of Neuropeptides. The fourth generation of progress. (www.acnp.org/g4GN401000047/CH.html), 2000

6. Golomb B and others. Severe irritability associated with statin cholesterol lowering drugs. *QJ Med.* 97:229-235. 2004.

CHAPTER 6 – Statins and Nuclear Factor *kappa*-B
1. Shovman O and others. Anti-inflammatory and immunomodulatory properties of statins. 2001
2. Hilgendorff A and others. Statins differ in their ability to block NF-kB activation in human blood monocytes. *Internat J Clin Pharm and Therapeut* 41(9): 397-401, 2003
3. Karin M, Delhase M. The 1 *kappa B* kinase and NF-*kappa B*: key elements of proinflammatory signaling. *Semin Immunol* 12(1): 85-98, 2000
4Masato E and others. Statins prevent tissue factor expression in human endothelial cells. *Circ* 103: 1736, 2002
5 Chen F and others. New insights into the role of nuclear factor kB in cell growth metabolism. *American Journal of Pathology* 159:387-397,2001
6. Karin M, Delhase M. The 1 *kappa B* kinase and NF-*kappa B*: key elements of proinflammatory signaling. *Semin Immunol* 12(1): 85-98, 2000
7. Tato CM and Hunter CM. Host-pathogen interactions: subversion and utilization of the NF-kB pathway during infection. *Infection and Immunity* 70(7): 3311-3317, 2002
8 . Raggatt LJ, Partridge NC. HMG-CoA reductase inhibitors as immunomodulators: potential use in transplant rejection. *Drugs* 62(15): 2185-91, 2002.
9. Kwak B and others. Statins as a newly recognized type of immunomodulator. *Nature Medicine* 6:1399-1402, 2000
10. Leung BP and others. A novel anti-inflammatory role for simvatatin in inflammatory arthritis. *J Immunol* 170(3): 1524-30, 2003
11.Palinski W. Immunomodulation: A new role for statins? *Nature Medicine* 6:1311-1312, 2000
12. Ravnskov U. *The Cholesterol Myths*, New Trends Publishing, 2000.
13. Rosch P. Statin drug side effects. *Proceeding of the Weston Price Foundation Meeting,* Spring 2003

14Matsuzaki M and others. Large-scale cohort study of the relationship between serum cholesterol concentration and coronary events with low-dose simvastatin therapy in Japanese patients with hypercholesterolemia. *Circ J* 66:1087-1095, 2002

CHAPTER 7 – The Role of Cholesterol in the Body.
1. Guyton AC, Hall JE. *The Adrenocortical Hormones.* In *Textbook of Medical Physiology*, 9th Ed, 957-971,Saunders, Philadelphia, 1996.
2. Russel DW. Green Light for Steroid Hormones. *Science* 272: 370-371, 1996.
3. Pfrieger F. Brain researcher discovers bright side of ill-famed molecule. *Science,* 9 November, 2001.
4. Pfrieger, F. Ibid.
5. Muldoon MF and others. Cholesterol Reduction and Non-Illness Mortality. Meta-Analysis of Randomized Clinical Trials. *British Medical Journal* 322: 11-15, 2001.
6. Golomb BA. Cholesterol and Violence: Is ThereConnection? *Annals of Internal Medicine* 128: 478-487, 1998.
7. Wolozin B and others. Decreased Prevalence of Alzheimer Disease Associated With 3-Hydroxy-3-MethyglutarylCoenzyme A Reduction Inhibitors. *Archives of Neurology* 57: 1439-1443, 2000.
8. Golomb B. Statins and Dementia. Letters to the Editor, *Archives of Neurology* 58(7), July 2001.
9. Pfrieger F. Cholesterol homeostasis and function in neurons of the central nervous system. *Cell Mol Life Sci* 60:1158-1171, 2003.
10. Lorin H. *Alzheimer's Solved.* Book Surge LLC, 2005
11. Kaplan M. Low Cholesterol Causes Aggressive.
12. Behavior and Depression. *Psychosomatic Medicine* 56: 479-484, 1994.
13. Bender KJ. *Psychiatric Times* 15(5), 1998.
14. Duits N, Bos F. Depressive Symptoms and Cholesterol Lowering Drugs. *Lancet* 341, Letter, 1999

181

15.Lechleitner M. Depressive Symptoms in Hypercholesterolaemic Patients Treated With Pravastatin, Letter, *Lancet* 340, Letter, 1999.
16. Buydens-Branchey L, Branchey M. Association between low plasma levels of cholesterol and relapse in cocaine addicts. *Psychosomatic Medicine* 65: 86-91, 2003.
17. Horwich TB and others. Low Serum totalcholesterol is associated with marked increase in mortality in advanced heart failure. *Journal of Cardiac Failure* 8(4), 2002.
18. McCully KS. *The Homocysteine Revolution.* Keats, 1997

CHAPTER 8 – Inflammation and Atherosclerosis
1. McCully KS. *The Homocysteine Revolution.* Keats, 1997
2. Pauling L. Unified Concept of Cardiovascular disease. http://www.ourhealthcoop.com/pauling.htm
3. McCully K. Homocysteine theory of arteriosclerosis: Development and current status. In Gotto AM, Paolett R, editors, *Atherosclerosis Reviews* 11: 157-246, Raven Press, New York, 1983.
4. McCully K. Atherosclerosis, serum cholesterol and the homocysteine theory: A study of 194 consecutive autopsies. *American Journal of the Medical Sciences* 299: 217-221, 1990.
5. Wilcken DE, Wilcken B. The pathogenesis of coronary heart disease. A possible role for methionine metabolism. *Journal of Clinical Investigation* 57: 1079-1082, 1976.
6. Boushey CJ and others. A quantitative assessment of plasma homocysteine as a risk factor for vascular disease. *Journal of the American Medical Association* 274: 1049-1057, 1995.
7. Kauffman J. Should you take aspirin to prevent heart attack? *Journal of Scientific Exploration* 14 (4): 623-641, 2000.
8. Ravnskov U. *The Cholesterol Myths*, New Trends Publishing, 2000.

CHAPTER 9 – The Misguided War on Cholesterol

1. Atkins, R. *Dr. Atkins' New Diet Revolution.* 3rd ed. Evans, New York, 2002.
2. Taubes G. What If It's All Been A Big, Fat Lie? *New York Times Magazine*, July 7, 2002.
3. Eades MR, Eades MD. *Protein Power.* Bantam Books, 1996.
4. Sears B. *The Zone.* Harper Collins, 1997.
5. Steward H and others. *Sugar Busters.* Ballentine Books, 1998.
6. McCully KS, McCully M. *The Heart Revolution.* Harper Collins, 2000.
7. Willett W. Turning The Food Pyramid Up Side Down. *American Journal of Clinical Nutrition* 76: 1261-1271, 2002.
8. Enig MG, Fallon S. The Mediterranean Diet--Pasta or Pastrami? *The Weston A. Price Foundation Magazine*, Spring, 2000.
9. ibid.
10.Keys A. Coronary heart disease in seven countries, *Circulation* 41(supplement 1), 1970.
11.Ibid.
12. Mann G. The great cholesterol scam. *21st centuryScience and Technology* 2(3), May-June 1989.

CHAPTER 10 – A Failed National Diet. What Diet, Then?
1. McCully KS, McCully M. *The Heart Revolution.* Harper Collins, 2000.
2. Banting, *Letter of Corpulence.* http://www.lowcarb.ca/corpulence/
3. Atkins RC. *Dr. Atkins' New Diet Revolution.* 3rd Ed. Evans, New York, 2002.
4. Kauffman J. Low carbohydrate diets. *Journal of Scientific Exploration,* 2004.
6. Braly J, Hoggan R. *Dangerous Grains: Why Gluten Cereal May Be Hazardous To Your Health.* Avery/Penguin Putnam, New York, 2002.
7. Ottoboni A, Ottoboni F. *The Modern Nutritional Diseases: Heart Disease, Stroke, Type-2 Diabetes, Obesity, Cancer,*

and How To Prevent Them. Vincenti Books, Sparks, NV, 2002.

8. McCully KS, McCully M. *The Heart Revolution.* Harper Collins, 2000.

9. Bernstein, R. *Dr. Bernstein's Diabetes Solution.* Little, Brown, Boston, 1997.

10. Smith MD. *Going Against the Grain: How Reducing and Avoiding Grains Can Revitalize Your Health.* Contemporary Books, Chicago, 2002.

11. Allan C, Lutz W. *Life Without Bread: How a Low-Carbohydrate Diet Can Save Your Life.* Keats, Los Angeles, 2000.

12. Groves B. *Eat Fat Get Thin.* Vermilion, London, 1999.

13. Eades MR, Eades MD. *The Protein Power Lifeplan.* Warner Books, New York, 2000.

14. Atkins RC. Dr. Atkins' *New Diet Revolution.* 3rd Ed. Evans, New York, 2002.

15. Kwasniewski MD, Chylinski M. *Homo Optimus.* Wydawnictwo WGP, Warsaw, 2000

16. Enig M, Fallon S. The Oiling of America. *Nexus Magazine*, Feb-Mar, 1999.

17. McCully KS, McCully M. *The Heart Revolution.* Harper Collins, 2000.

18. Fallon S, Enig M. What causes heart disease? Lancet 1: 1062-1065, 1983

19. Kauffman J. Should you take aspirin to prevent heart attack? *Journal of Scientific Exploration* 14 (4): 623-641, 2000.

CHAPTER 11- Enter Glyconutrients

1. Kidd P. *Altern Med Rev* 5(1):16, 2000

2. Hsu HY and others. *Am J Chin Med* 18 (1-2):61-69,1990

3. Pande and Kuman M. *Pharmaceut Biol* 36(3):227-232, 1998

4. Eggar SF and others. *Cancer Immunol Immunother* 43(4):195-205, 1996

5. Matsunaga K and others. *Invasion Metastasiks* 16(1): 27-38, 1996

6. Matsunaga K and others. *Oncology* 51(4):303-308, 1994
7. Saavedra J and others. *J Pediatr Gastroenterol Nutr* 29(4):95A, 1999
8. Saavedra J and others. *J Pediatr Gastroenterol Nutr* 29(4):58A, 1999
9. Arcadi VC. *Dynamic Chiropractic* February 26, 1996
10. M. Vander-Wal, C.E. Pippenger, *Proc. Fish. Inst. Med. Res.*, 3 (2); 9-12, 2004.
11. Watson M. *Arthritis Rheum* 42(8):1682-90, 1999

CHAPTER 12 - Anti-Inflammatory Alternatives to Statins

1.Langsjoen P, Langsjoen E. Statin associated congestive heart failure. *Proceedings of Weston-Price Foundation Meeting*, Spring, 2003.
2. Langsjoen P, Langsjoen A. Coenzyme Q10 In cardiovascular disease with emphasis on heart failure and myocardial ischemia. *Asia Pacific Heart Journal* 7(3): 160-168, 1998.
3. Bargossi AM and others. Exogenous CoQ10 supplementation prevents ubiquinone reduction induced by HMG- CoA reductase inhibitors. *Mol Aspects Med.* 15(Suppl): S187-93, 1994 4. De Pinieux and others. Lipid-lowering drugs and mitochondrial function: effects of HMG-CoA reductase inhibitors on serum ubiquinone and blood lactate/pyruvate ratio. *Br J Clin Pharmacol.* 42(3): 333-37, 1996
5. Ely JTA, Krone CA. A brief update on ubiquinone (Coenzyme Q10). *J Orthomol Med* 15(2): 63-8, 2000
6.Ely JTA, Krone CA. Urgent update on ubiquinone (Coenzyme Q10), 2000 (www.faculty.washington.edu/ely/turnover.html)
7. Wallace DC. Mitochondrial DNA in aging and disease, *Sci Amer;* 40-7, 1997
8.Pauling L. Unified theory of heart disease. 1991 http://www.ourhealthcoop.com/pauling.htm
9. Lee KW, Lip GYH. The Role of Omega-3 in the Secondary Prevention of Cardiovascular Disease. *Quarterly Journal of Medicine* 96: 465-480, 2003.

10 Omega-3 information service http://www.omega-3info.com/home.htm

11 Covington M. Omega-3 fatty acids. *AFP* 70(1) July 2004

12McCully KS. The Homocysteine Revolution. Keats,1997.

13.Ubbink JB, *American Journal of Clinical Nutrition*, Jan 1993;57: 47-53

14. Selhub J and others. *JAMA* 270:2693-2698, 1993

15.Naurath HJ and others. *Lancet* 346:85-91, 1995

16 . Kauffman J. *Malignant Medical Myths*. Infinity Publishing, 2005

17.Matsuzaki M and others. Large scale cohort study of the relationship between serum cholesterol concentration and coronary events with low-dose simvastatin therapy in Japanese patients with hypercholesterolemia. *Circ J* 66:1087-1095, 2002

18.Hilgendorff A and others. Statins differ in their ability to block NF-kB activation in human blood monocytes. *Internat J Clin Pharm Therapeut* 41(9): 397-401, 2003

19. Law MR and others. Quantifying effect of statins on low density lipoprotein cholesterol, ischaemic heart disease, and stroke: systematic review and meta-analysis. *BMJ* 326:1423, 2006

20.Shovman O and others. Anti-inflammatory and Immunomodulatory properties of statins. *Immunol Res* 25(3): 272-85, 2002

21. Heber D and others. Cholesterol lowering effects of a proprietary Chinese red yeast rice dietary supplement.*American Journal of Clinical Nutrition 69:* 231-236, 1999.

22. Tan, B. and A. M. Mueller. Tocotrienols in Cardiometabolic Diseases. *Tocotrienols:Vitamin E beyond Tocopherol*. R. Watson, AOCS Press. 2008.

23. Peskin, B and Habib A. *The Hidden Story of Cancer*. Pinnacle Press. 2008

CHAPTER 13. Failure of MedWatch

1.http://www.spacedoc.net/662_cases_memory_loss

CHAPTER 14. Serious Statin Drug Statin Side Effects
a)The ALS/Statin Link

1. Meske V and others. *European Journal of Neuroscience.* 17: 93, 2003

2. Lambourne S and others. *Molecular and Cellular Biology,* 2005 http://mcb.asm.org/cgi/content/abstract/25/1/278

3. Ferrer I. and others, *Current Alzheimer's Research,* 2005 http://mcb.asm.org/cgi/content/abstract/25/1/278

4. Sharma N and Lee M. Two to tangle: the story of *tau* Eukaryon 1:28-32, 2006

5. Mathuranath P. *Tau* and tauopathies. 55(1) 11-16, 2007
Statins and ALS-Like Syndrome

b.) Permanent Peripheral Neuropathy
1. Jospeh Tuazon, PharmD. Medical Information Manager, Pfizer U.S. Medical Information. NDA (New Drug Application) studies. Changes in Memory and Cogition with Tables 1&2. Pfizer Inc. 182 Tabor Road, Morris Plains, NJ 07950 14 June 2006
c.) Permanent Myopathy
1. Vladutiu G and others. Genetic risk factors associated with lipid-lowering drug-induced myopathies. *Muscle Nerve* 34: 153-162, 2006

2. Golomb BA, Evans, MA 2008. Statin Adverse Effects: A Review of the Literature & Evidence for a Mitochondrial Mechanism. *American Journal of Cardiovascular Drugs.* March 2009, (in press)

d.) Chronic Neuromuscular Degeneration
1. Draeger and others. Statin therapy induces ultrastructural damage in skeletal muscle in patients without myalgia. *Pathology* 210: 94-102, 2002
2. Caso G and others. Statin therapy induces ultrastructural damage in skeletal muscle in patients without myalgia. Journal of Pathology 210: 94-102, 2006
3. Campbell W. Statin myopathy: The iceberg or its tip? *Muscle & Nerve* 34(4): 387-390, 2006
4. Vladutiu G and others. Genetic risk factors associated with lipid-lowering drug-induced myopathies. Muscle Nerve 34: 153-162, 2006
5. Mooseman B and Behl C. Selenoprotein synthesis and side effects of statins. *Lancet* 363:892-94, 2004

CHAPTER 15. Mitochondrial Mutations
1. Mooseman B and Behl C. Selenoprotein synthesis and side effects of statins. Lancet 363:892-94, 2004
2. http://www.ncbi.nlm.nih.gov/pubmed/18606916
3. *American Journal of Clinical Nutrition*, Vol. 88, No. 3, 801-809, September 2008
4. http://www.ncbi.nlm.nih.gov/pubmed/18606916